D1598670

THE VOICE OF BREAST CANCER IN MEDICINE AND BIOETHICS

Philosophy and Medicine

VOLUME 88

The titles published in this series are listed at the end of this volume

THE VOICE OF BREAST CANCER IN MEDICINE AND BIOETHICS

Edited by

MARY C. RAWLINSON

Stony Brook University, Stony Brook, NY, U.S.A.

and

SHANNON LUNDEEN

University of Pennsylvania, Philadelphia, PA, U.S.A.

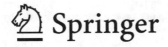 Springer

A C.I.P. Catalogue record for this book is available from the Library of Congress.

ISBN-10 1-4020-4508-5 (HB)
ISBN-13 978-1-4020-4508-0 (HB)
ISBN-10 1-4020-4477-1 (e-book)
ISBN-13 978-1-4020-4477-9 (e-book)

Published by Springer,
P.O. Box 17, 3300 AA Dordrecht, The Netherlands.

www.springer.com

Printed on acid-free paper

Printed in the Netherlands.

TABLE OF CONTENTS

ACKNOWLEDGEMENTS

This book grew out of a conference on breast cancer sponsored by the Program in Women's Studies at Stony Brook University in 2002. Professors Sherwin, Lerner, Kovach, Diedrich, and Lobel participated in the conference which was organized by Helen Rodnite Lemay and Mary C. Rawlinson.

The editors would like to thank Lisa Rasmussen, the Managing Editor of the Philosophy and Medicine book series, for her generous support and assistance in bringing the volume to publication.

INTRODUCTION

ROSEMARIE TONG

NEGOTIATING PERSONAL AND POLITICAL SETTLEMENTS WITH BREAST CANCER

Women Finding Their Own Ways to Live with Human Contingency

Yesterday as I was pushing my shopping cart up and down the aisles of the grocery store, my eyes glanced over to the tabloid rack. I immediately noticed that the feature story in the *Globe* was an exclusive interview entitled "Jacklyn Smith Wins Battle with Breast Cancer" (*Globe* 2003). Making sure no one I know saw me, I plunked my money down for the scandal sheet and took it home where my prurient interests got the best of me. I read the whole issue, although I had initially planned to read only the Jacklyn Smith story. Not surprisingly, Smith's breast-cancer story had a familiar plot line. Her narrative began with her fears about disfigurement and even death; progressed to her "courageous" decision to consent to a lumpectomy with subsequent radiation; and ended with a radiant (and very sexy) Jacklyn Smith holding up her "clean bill of health" as she returned full force to her work and relationships. Why, I wondered, is the *Globe* making it sound as if Smith's experience is somehow extraordinary and exceptional, when 220,000 new cases of breast cancer in the U.S. were reported in 2002 alone? Far from being unique, Jacklyn Smith's story is increasingly the one many breast-cancer patients tell. And yet, despite the fact that more women are living well with breast cancer than dying badly from it, American women continue to fear breast cancer much more than the actual number one killer of American women: cardiac disease.

In large measure, this anthology, skillfully assembled by philosophers Mary Rawlinson and Shannon Lundeen, explains the many reasons why breast cancer in particular continues to occupy U.S. women's attention. In the lead essay, philosopher Susan Sherwin addresses the politics of cancer in her probing chapter entitled "Personalizing the Political: Negotiating Feminist, Medical, Scientific, and Commercial Discourses Surrounding Breast Cancer." Sherwin begins by highlighting the "dualisms" that characterize breast-cancer debates; it's largely

ix

genetically-determined...no, it's mostly environmentally-produced; it's being cured...no, it's on the rise; be a cheerful cancer patient with a smiley face...no, be a realistic cancer patient with eyes wide open; and so on. Sherwin's multiperspectival analysis of breast cancer is informed by her feminist sensitivities. In particular, her thoughts are guided by the omnipresent question, "Who benefits and who is harmed by the existing policies?" Is it women with breast cancer? Or is it researchers who want to be famous; pharmaceutical companies who want to increase profits; and/or politicians who want to be elected?

Sherwin reminds us that in the 1970s women helped politicize the personal—in this instance, the very personal experience of breast cancer. Among others, Shirley Temple Black, Happy Rockefeller, and Betty Ford told their breast-cancer stories in public. They thereby encouraged women to bring the breast cancer they had hidden in their bedrooms and bathrooms out into the public domain. Soon thousands of women were talking to each other and to anyone else who would listen about their disease. Various segments of the public started to "racing" for the cure, participating in fundraising marathons and lobbying Congress for higher breast-cancer-research appropriations. Women were urged to self-exam their breasts and to get mammograms on an annual basis. Breast-cancer support groups multiplied, and, eventually, a whole month was devoted to increasing breast cancer awareness. But breast cancer's acceptance into the public domain was not without its problems. Sherwin observes that cancer became so political that many women felt that their own breast cancer—their own personal worries and pains—had to be experienced in a certain way. Sherwin claims that two metaphors—that of breast cancer as an enemy against whom war must be waged, and that of women's bodies as the terrain on which the enemy advances—created a framework of "danger, urgency, and fear" (p. 12). Women were expected to fight the enemy with the weapons in medicine's arsenal. To fail to fight the enemy to the finish was to be viewed as either a crazy woman or a coward.

While recognizing the role of biomedical tools in arresting breast cancer's assault on women's bodies, Sherwin notes that the breast-cancer establishment has focused on surgery, radiotherapy, chemotherapy, and pharmacotherapy without exploring in any real depth other ways to treat breast cancer, some of which may be found in the annals of alternative and complementary medicine, for example. Nor has the breast-cancer establishment, at least of late, focused enough attention on the possible environmental causes of breast cancer. Could it be that there is more money to be made and fame to be had in finding a spectacular cure for breast cancer than in quietly preventing its inception? In other words, could it be that it is more glamorous to wage war on an acute disease than to make peace with a chronic disease—to live as well as one can with it?

Sherwin encourages each woman who has breast cancer to feel free to "depoliticize" her breast cancer and to come to terms with it in her own unique way. It is not irrational for a breast-cancer victim to refuse radiotherapy and/or chemotherapy; nor is it weird for her to refuse breast reconstruction subsequent to breast-cancer surgery. Different people have different priorities and values, and these differences produce different ways of being ill and different strategies for negotiating the challenges of breast cancer.

The second chapter, "Power, Gender, and Pizzazz: The Early Years of Breast Cancer Activism," by the historian Barron H. Lerner, who is both an M.D. and a Ph.D., provides a telling account of four breast-cancer victims who became breast-cancer activists (Babette Rosmond, Rose Kushner, Betty Rollin, and Audre Lorde). Each of these *activist* victims played an important role in convincing both patients and physicians that each woman who experiences breast cancer must write her own breast-cancer journal, accepting and rejecting treatments as she sees fit. Rosmond's and Kushner's activism took the form of furthering the patients' rights agenda, emphasizing the importance of securing women's *informed consent* to breast-cancer treatments, therapies, and drugs. Rosmond encouraged women to take charge of their disease; to find out for themselves its nature and consequences; and to look for physicians, including path-breaking researchers, able and willing to treat them in the way they wanted to be treated. Specifically, in her own case, Rosmond was convinced that there had to be a better way to treat breast cancer than the standard of care for breast cancer in her time; namely, the unnecessarily mutilating radical mastectomy (removal of not only the cancerous breast and adjacent lymph nodes but also the chest wall muscles on both sides of the cancer). Her conviction turned out to be true. There was a better standard of care for her kind of breast cancer. Thanks to physicians Oliver Cope and especially George Crile, Jr., partial mastectomy (most usually lumpectomy), followed (or not followed) by radiotherapy and, in some instances, also chemotherapy is currently the general recommendation for women with small cancers.

No doubt, the results of Rosmond's efforts, published in book form as *The Invisible Worm*, helped motivate Rose Kushner to demand even more. Kushner saw no reason to automatically permit physicians to engage in a so-called one-step approach to breast cancer ("I'll do a biopsy, and if things look bad, I'll do what I think is best for you right on the spot"). On the contrary, she insisted that, ordinarily, there should be a two-step approach to breast cancer ("I'll do a biopsy, and, then, later you'll decide what kind of surgery is best for you"). So feisty was Kushner, a journalist by trade, that she chided First Lady Betty Ford in 1974 for agreeing to a one-step radical mastectomy in the event her biopsy showed cancer. She thought Ford was setting a bad example for women, and she told her so. As Kushner saw it, women had a responsibility not only to learn as much as possible about breast cancer but also to remain actively in control of their treatment at all times. A rather heavy responsibility, when one thinks about it; and perhaps one that women should feel free *not* to bear!

Although Rollin and Lorde also focused on breast-cancer treatment issues, some of their most interesting contributions to the breast-cancer debate honed in on issues related to women's appearance. Rollin, a television correspondent for NBC News, who authored a book entitled *First You Cry*, reassured women with breast cancer that it was neither crazy nor wrong for them to express concerns about their looks before they started to focus on their health. In fact, Rollin confessed that, in her own case of breast cancer, she was for a time fixated on whether she could ever wear a strapless dress again. She viewed as utterly uncaring the physician who recommended that, subsequent to breast-cancer surgery, women should "stuff an old stocking" in their bra and get on with life matter-of-factly. Rollin observed that such a recommendation is hard for women to follow in a society that fetishizes women's breasts as the primary sign and symbol of their physical attractiveness and, to a lesser extent, reproductive health. Even women who know better, who do not want to be reduced to their bodies and judged only in terms of their beauty, sometimes worry about their "cup size" (is it A, B, C, D, E?), and whether their "too-big" or "too-little" breasts are somehow detracting from their desirability as women.

Disagreeing with Rollin, Lorde in her *Cancer Journals* imposed a heavy duty on women who regard themselves as feminists. Despite the fact that she mourned the loss of her breast, which had been one of the sites of pleasure for her and her lesbian partner, Lorde advised women not to have breast reconstruction subsequent to breast-cancer surgery. Lorde felt pressured by health care professionals to fix-up her unsightly chest which, to them, apparently constituted an unnecessary eyesore. They could not understand why a woman would not want breast reconstruction. After all, it would make her "whole" again! To this line of reasoning, Lorde objected that she, Audre Lorde, was far more than her body, and certainly far more than a *part* of her body—namely, her breast. Rather than "repairing" her loss, she would wear it as a sign that the powers-that-be had failed her and other women by not doing enough to prevent breast cancer. If Lorde was going to cry about anything, it would be her health, and not her appearance.

In the third chapter, Gwynne Gertz provides us with a history of the medical discourse surrounding breast cancer and breast cancer treatment. Like Sherwin, Gertz points to the way in which breast cancer treatment methods have been informed by a predominantly militaristic discourse that treats the woman's body as a battlefield and the cancer as the enemy that must be annihilated. More than supporting the highly invasive Halsted radical mastectomy as the superlative form of treatment, the predominance of militaristic tropes in physicians' discussions of breast cancer research actually worked to determine the validity of new developments in breast cancer treatment. Employing Bakhtin's language theory, Gertz explains how this traditional medical discourse eventually became "interilluminated" with the voices of patients and physicians who challenged the effectiveness of all-out surgical wars on the bodies of women with breast disease. Together, these patients and the physicians who listened to them, worked to disclose the effectiveness and scientific validity of less-invasive breast cancer treatment methods.

Lisa Diedrich's paper also offers a critique of the dominant discourse of breast cancer. She observes that, in the framework of the biomedical view of cancer, both patients' and physicians' roles are limited. In particular, she notes "what is expected, even required, of persons who are ill is that they perform a passively heroic mode of being ill, while their doctors perform an actively heroic mode of curing" (p. 54). Diedrich then compares Susan Sontag's and Eve Kosofsky Sedgwick's very different ways of defying the biomedical view of cancer, and of dealing with not only breast cancer but also HIV-AIDS on their own terms.

Diedrich reminds her readers that, as women, Sontag and Sedgwick both experienced breast cancer in their own lives, with all the requisite fears and pains associated with it; but, as writers and thinkers, they chose to present the disease differently to readers. According to Diedrich, Sontag decided to challenge the way illness is experienced and narrativized by doing things with *ideas*, while Sedgwick decided to achieve the same goal by doing things with *affects* (p. 55).

In her book, *Illness as Metaphor*, Sontag emphasizes how metaphors can hurt people with a disease by convincing them their disease has a moral meaning, or is somehow a mandatory call to make their lives more meaningful. She claims the most effective way to deal with disease is not to let it into one's imagination, where it will play all sorts of games, many of them hurtful, but instead to coolly conceptualize the disease so it can be reduced to an idea one can intellectually control. Several years after writing *Illness as Metaphor*, HIV-AIDS entered Sontag's circle of friends as well as the public at large. When this happened, Sontag acknowledged the "panic and animal terror" she initially felt when she was diagnosed with breast cancer and used ideas to tame her fears (and shame) about it. She also confessed some growing doubts about the advisability of continuing to approach disease dispassionately and draining it of its metaphorical content. However, as Diedrich sees it, Sontag's moments of doubt were not frequent enough to help her clearly see that although some disease metaphors like "cancer personality" are damaging and debilitating, other disease metaphors like "cancer survivor" may have beneficial consequences. It is not necessarily wrong to give disease a moral meaning—not if this meaning has liberating effects.

Diedrich contrasts Sontag's way of managing disease with Sedgwick's. According to Diedrich, the ability to engage Sedgwick's concept of "queer performativity" can help people with diseases like breast cancer and HIV-AIDS deal with their disease as *whole* persons—that is, as people with minds in which concrete images and abstract ideas, emotions and ratiocinations continually intersect, begging for the relief only a story about one's self-meaning can provide.

Diedrich explains that for Sedgwick "queer" is a "continuing movement across bodies and differences. It is at once relational—it perceives beings in relation—and strange—it doesn't attempt to make anyone's gender or sexuality 'signify monolithically'" (p. 62). Being—doing "queer"—permits people to experience their own breast cancer or HIV-AIDS in relation to their multiple selves (e.g., the fearful self, the hopeful self, the old healthy self, the new unhealthy self, the self that may yet be) and to connect with other selves who have multiple personae. To do breast cancer "queerly" is to "out" it and include others in one's experience. Rather than hiding one's disease and keeping it private, or seeking to control one's disease by reducing it to an idea with no emotional content, queerness induces people "to entrust as many people as one possibly can with one's actual body and its needs, one's stories about its fate, one's dreams and one's sources of information or hypothesis about disease, cure, consolation, denial, and the state or institutional violence that are also invested in one's illness" (p. 65, quoting Sedgwick). Life lived under the rubric "Out, out" and "Include, include" instead of the rubric "In, in" and "Exclude, exclude" is full of possibilities for the self, even in the throes of disease and in view of impending death.

In the second section of the volume, "Narratives of Breast Cancer: Living with Disease," we are presented with illuminating reflections on living with breast disease. Each author in this section, whether writing about themselves or others with breast cancer, documents the struggle of *how to be with others* in the face of such an illness. In the first chapter, Anita Ho, a professor of philosophy who specializes in feminist bioethics, details her efforts to reconcile her academic training with her experiences of being diagnosed with and treated for breast cancer. Through her diary entries we find that Ho's bout with breast cancer forces her to encounter first-hand the problems with the healthcare system that she had been teaching her students about in her bioethics courses. From fragmented treatment to neglect in obtaining informed consent for medical procedures to having her breasts treated as independent from the rest of her body—Ho's diary entries demonstrate how the health care system itself may contribute to the patient's suffering. .

Not only does Ho have to figure out how best to negotiate a fragmented healthcare system in deciding the most appropriate treatment for her breast disease, but she also has to renegotiate her personal relationships. The physical effects of undergoing treatments for breast cancer force Ho to come to terms with the extent to which her identity as a heterosexual woman is informed by certain standards of femininity. Disarmed by the physical appearance of her chest post-treatment, Ho observes that, "It is ironic that I am unable to defy the culture that I try to convince my students to reject. I feel embarrassed that, at the moment of truth, I have succumbed to the breast culture. I sometimes stand in front of the mirror, trying to find ways to correct the lopsidedness of my breasts. I refuse to let Carl look at my scarred and burned breast, worrying that his desire for me will diminish" (p. 88).

Ho's narrative provides substantive examples of the claims that feminist bioethicists have made about approaches to women's health in our healthcare system: namely, that fragmented health care results in a patient's lack of access to information about her body and her treatment and an overall feeling of helplessness in this regard, that there are problems with the procedures for obtaining informed consent, that the fragmentation of the female body in the name of "treatment" has pernicious effects on the bodily integrity of a patient, and that the healthcare system often fails to acknowledge the psychological struggles that women go through to maintain/regain a healthy, positive body image in the face of debilitating illnesses and/or treatments.

In "Breast Cancer: The Maternal Body Reflected in a Three-way Mirror," psychologist and psychoanalyst Debra Gold powerfully recounts the way in which breast cancer has *literally* shaped her relationships with her mother and her daughter. Gold's essay reveals the extent to which a mother-daughter relationship is wrought with physical assumptions about the maternal body; assumptions that are undermined and challenged by a mother with breast cancer. Not only are the presuppositions regarding the shape, look, and feel of the maternal body contested by physically-altering breast cancer treatments, but so too are the notions of a mother's touch and propinquity. In this essay, Gold guides us through the delicate terrain of coming to terms with the myriad ways in which cross-generational breast cancer has reshaped not only the bodies of those it has dwelt in, but their most intimate relationships as well.

Leatha Kendrick's chapter, "Learn to Love What's Left—Poems of Breast Cancer," is comprised of a set of poems all detailing different stages of living with breast cancer and undergoing treatment for it. Taking us from her diagnosis, through her treatments, and to her hopes for survival post-mastectomy, Kendrick's poems reconcile her body before breast cancer with "what's left" after her treatment. By the end of the last poem in her chapter, we get the sense that, although she still harbors a fear that the cancer may return, Kendrick has learned to love herself anew.

In "Death and the Other: Rethinking Authenticity," feminist phenomenologist Gail Weiss argues, contra philosopher Martin Heidegger, that when faced with a potentially terminal illness such as breast cancer, not only must we share experiences of being-toward-death with others, but that public narratives of such experiences are authentic descriptions of being-toward-death. Weiss reads journalist Cathy Hainer's public breast cancer journals (published in *USA TODAY* 1998-1999 just before her death) as issuing a compelling challenge to Heidegger's description of authenticity in being-toward-death.

Heidegger's analysis of Dasein's being-toward-death suggests that facing death involves being alone, accepting death as *mine,* and accepting it as that part of the human condition that involves being radically broken off from others. Weiss describes Hainer's engagement with others in facing her death: "As Cathy anticipates her death, contemplating the transformation of its indefinite certainty to a definite one, she receives her greatest pleasures from the affection and love she gives and receives with her family and friends" (p. 108). Whereas Heidegger's analysis of being-toward-death suggests that our relationships with others become undone, Hainer's journals, as well as the narratives presented by the other authors in this section of the volume, suggest that facing one's own fatality demands intimacy with others through which the distance between oneself and others is traversed (p. 111). Heidegger also characterizes as necessarily inauthentic any musings on one's being-toward-death in a public forum—such as that of an international newspaper. However, Weiss maintains that public accounts, such as Hainer's, not only authentically describe one's being-toward-death, but help us to make sense of "the relationship between death and the other" by revealing such unique experiences in familiar and accessible language against the backdrop of an otherwise mundane and familiar life (p. 112).

In the opening essay of the third section of the volume, "Breast Cancer as a Model in Clinical Research" physician John S. Kovach invites the public, politicians, and scientists "to partner in prioritizing projects and resources" so as "to reduce the burden of life-threatening chronic diseases" (p. 119) such as breast cancer. Kovach highlights failures as well as successes in breast-cancer research. As he sees it, bad research occurs when special interest groups pressure scientists to look for evidence that supports their political causes. For example, in the 1980s a set of twelve breast-cancer studies, collectively known as the Long Island Breast Cancer Study Project (LIBCSP), were conducted. The thirty million dollar project was undertaken primarily because breast cancer advocates in the Northeast were convinced that PAHs (combustion products of fossil fuels and tobacco) were responsible for the high rates of cancer in certain Northeast locations. When the first two studies in the costly project did not find a significant correlation between presence of PAHs in the environment and high cancer rates, critics of the Project implied that the government had wasted thirty million dollars on the LIBCSP project merely because fear-mongering activists had (falsely) convinced Long Islanders that PAHs were *the* enemy to fight in the war against breast cancer. The critics then further implied that had Long Islanders not been misled by environmentalists and women's health zealots, they would not have pressured for fruitless studies, and scientists could have instead used government monies to do better cancer studies. However, Kovach points out that even if the LIBCSP project did not prove what it set out to prove, it is still very likely that environmental factors like the presence of PAHs probably do contribute to high cancer rates, but in very complex ways that involve an intricate interplay between environmental factors and genetically-determined propensities to certain kinds of cancer in particular populations. A scientific optimist, Kovach predicts that cancer-research projects will improve as scientists learn how to resist inappropriate and unrealistic political pressures and to instead work with politicians and the public to conduct the kind of research that is likely to really serve their health-related interests.

Loretta Kopelman's chapter, "Clinical Trials for Breast Cancer and Informed Consent: How Women Helped Make Research a Cooperative Endeavor," reinforces the notion that breast-cancer patients should actively partner with clinicians as well as researchers/investigators in the treatment of their disease. As Kopelman sees it, for decades clinicians and investigators/researchers operated on the paternalistic assumption that women with breast cancer could not understand the best treatment options for their disease, let alone the advisability of entering (or not entering) a randomized clinical trial (RCT). Because of this misguided view and the belief that Halsted's radical mastectomy was *the* standard of care for treating breast cancer, most clinicians did not even present women with the option of entering a RCT. But then women began doing their own research about breast cancer. They discovered that some researchers/investigators were developing relatively non-disfiguring treatments for breast cancer, and that they needed research subjects to prove the safety and efficacy of them. Gradually, patients, clinicians, and researchers/investigators developed an approach to RCTs that served their intersecting interests; but the path to this successful conclusion was not without some major hurdles due to the design of a typical RCT.

When a patient's life is at stake, and she enters a RCT in which she may be assigned to either the group of patients who receive the standard of care treatment (in the "old days," the radical mastectomy) or the group of patients who receive the promising, but by no means "sure-bet" experimental treatment (lumpectomy in this scenario), patients' and clinicians' anxiety levels are likely to be high. Patients will demand adequate information about the true risks and benefits of the RCT before they sign on the dotted line; and clinicians will seek reassurance from researchers/investigators that their patients will be helped, or at least not harmed by participating in the RCT. Thus, researchers/investigators may be tempted to stress the benefits and downplay the risks of their RCTs in an attempt to get enough patients to enroll in them and enough clinicians to endorse them.

Because of the state of affairs described above, RCTs were trapped in a vicious ethical circle for a long time. Kopelman summarizes the dilemma as follows:

> If rigorous consent is sought for RCTs, then the likelihood increases that biases will be introduced as (1) distinct groups favor particular treatments, (2) accrual rate will be slow, (3) some may drop out. Any of these circumstances could affect the reliability of the RCT or create problems for the analysis of the data. But if one undermines the integrity of RCTs then arguably it is better not to conduct them. (p. 144)

This vicious ethical circle was broken by developing several new RCT designs, each of which was able to provide for true informed consent.

While more studies need to be conducted on the genetic and environmental causes of breast cancer, Anne Moyer and Marci Lobel demonstrate in their chapter, "The Role of Psychosocial Research in Understanding and Improving the Experience of Breast Cancer and Breast Cancer Risk" that studies of the psychosocial effects of breast cancer on patients are also crucially important. Moyer and Lobel are particularly concerned about the ways in which women at risk for breast cancer (for example, with a family history of the disease) overestimate the chances that they will actually suffer from the disease, and what, if anything, can and should be done about this risk misperception. In a measured way, Moyer and Lobel discuss some at-risk women's decisions to undergo bilateral prophylactic mastectomy even when others deem such surgery as unwarranted. Contrary to common lore, most women who decide on this dramatic course of action do not live to regret their decision—at least that is what follow-up studies show (p. 165).

Among the most interesting topics Moyer and Lobel discuss are studies that point to which techniques are most promising in reducing breast-cancer patients' nausea and vomiting during the course of chemotherapy. The expectation of the symptom may produce the symptom, and therapists should try to use their skills to prevent patients from talking themselves into feeling queasy (pp. 129-130). However, while recognizing the importance pf psychological factors, Moyer and Lobel are quick to note that recent research calls into question the previously posited link between a "fighting spirit" and positive outcomes in terms of cancer recurrence and survival. Such a spirit—however admirable—appears to be neither a necessary nor a sufficient condition for living longer or better with cancer. Moyer and Lobel also make it clear that breast cancer patients need not fear saying "no" to participation in a support group. Studies show, say Moyer and Lobel, that one-on-one educational interventions are just as likely if not more likely than group therapy sessions to give breast cancer patients a sense of control over their disease. Indeed, some women with breast cancer are harmed by support group experiences, finding them a site for "uncomfortable or fear-arousing topics" (p. 171). The best part of Moyer and Lobel's total honest recitation of current psychosocial research about breast cancer is the last section on end-of-life issues. Rather than "sugar-coating" the last days of the lives of women with metastatic breast cancer, Moyer and Lobel admit there is often a "significant elevation in mood disturbance, symptoms of trauma, and pain" conjoined with "a decrease in the ability to experience positive states of mind" (p. 174). Dying from advanced breast cancer is no easier than dying from any other disease that methodically breaks one's body down as it pushes through the dying process.

In the last section of this anthology, "Breast Cancer in the Classroom," we are presented with the works of a Distinguished Teaching Professor, Helen Rodnite Lemay and two students, one graduate student and one undergraduate, who worked with Lemay in a program on women's health. In her chapter, "Teaching About Breast Cancer and 'Common Health,'" Helen Rodnite Lemay describes how she used a course on HIV-AIDS to construct a university Women and Medicine course with a several-week-long segment on breast cancer. The general aim of the course was to help students replace the concept of health as an individual state with the concept of health as a communal, *common* human quality. Lemay sought to implement the course's aim by first showing her students how many diseases, including breast cancer, are continually culturally restructured through history. Specifically, she showed her students how the symbolic meaning of women's breasts has changed over time. The breasts, once viewed as objects of worship by fertility cults, gradually became objects of erotic arousal for men in particular.

As the course went on, Lemay and her students discussed how women's breasts are not only symbols of women's reproductive and sexual roles but also sources of profit for several industries and professions. Lemay and her students became somewhat disheartened as they "learned about the close ties between medical politics and the development of biometrics, radiation and the modified radical mastectomy"; and as they "realized just how interested members of the male medical guild were in professional advancement, and how heavily this weighed in their choice of treatment for women patients" (pp. 179-180).

Lemay and her class went on to uncover instances in which corporations exaggerate claims of benefit in order to promote their breast-cancer projects. They pondered the case of a pharmaceutical company that sponsored a Breast Cancer Awareness month program. The company, which produces herbicides and pesticides, allegedly censored printed material that described environmental causes of breast cancer. Instead, the company focused on an individual-based rather than community-based action plan to combat the disease, including mammography and other costly examinations.

Among the lessons Lemay and her class took to heart were those about how individual women with breast cancer find themselves situated among discordant choices of whether, and how, to select treatment. She and her students discussed the dilemmas of women who refused breast-cancer treatment because they were pregnant (metaphors of sainthood and martyrdom were common). In addition, they discussed how easy it is to politicize the personal decision of whether to go through breast reconstruction; and how regrettable it is when women, who should be comforting each other through the breast-cancer experience, instead fight with each other about the "politically correct" or "true feminist" reaction to a disfigured body.

Although I am tempted to describe in detail other important lessons Lemay and her class learned—lessons about the ways in which one's race and class affect breast cancer rates, awareness, and reactions as well as lessons about the ways in which breast-cancer activism can be "bad" as "good"—I will restrain myself from doing so. Instead, I am going to seriously consider developing a course, modeled on Lemay's course, at my own university. I am convinced that courses such as Lemay's can help many women live well with breast cancer, and, when the time for living is over, die well with cancer.

Certainly, the two papers by Lemay's students demonstrate the positive results of focusing on breast cancer in the classroom. In her essay "Theoretical Considerations on 'Reading' the Breast," Tanfer Emin-Tunc reflects on the work of a reading group on breast cancer which she organized under Lemay's direction. Emin-Tunc makes a compelling argument for the role of feminist epistemology in understanding and coping with breast cancer. She shows how helping students develop a critical approach can move them beyond the merely anecdotal and personal to a consideration of the cultural context in which the female body is represented, as well as the public policies through which it is approached. Sofya Maslyanskaya's "Recent Developments in Breast Cancer Research," is a direct response to Dr. Kovach's chapter. Maslyanskaya expands upon Kovach's essay and documents recent developments in breast cancer research. Maslyanskaya's interest in women's health took her beyond the undergraduate classroom and into medical school at the State University of New York Downstate where she is currently a second-year medical student.

Mary Rawlinson and Shannon Lundeen are to be heartily applauded for constructing an anthology on breast cancer in which a set of essays actually fit together and tell a compelling story not only about women's pain and suffering but also women's strength, resilience, and courage. Although the voices and perspectives expressed in the anthology are very different, their overall message is the same. It is one of self-reflectiveness, cooperation, and serving women's best interests.

Rosemarie Tong is Distinguished Professor of Health Care Ethics and Director of the Center for Professional and Applied Ethics at the University of North Carolina at Charlotte. She is the Co-Coordinator of the International Feminist Approaches to Bioethics Network.

REFERENCES

Globe. 2003. Jacklyn Smith wins battle with breast cancer. September, 9: 6-7.

I. Discourses of Breast Cancer: Who Speaks for Breast Cancer?

CHAPTER ONE

SUSAN SHERWIN

PERSONALIZING THE POLITICAL

Negotiating Feminist, Medical, Scientific, and Commercial Discourses
Surrounding Breast Cancer

1. INTRODUCTION: DIFFERENT TAKES ON BREAST CANCER

What do we now know about breast cancer? The answer largely depends on whom you ask. There are currently many lively debates about many aspects of breast cancer with authoritative proponents on different sides of most issues. Consider the following dualisms. In most cases, the first element represents the most common thinking about breast cancer and the second represents a critical alternative.

- Breast cancer is curable if detected early. Breast cancer can be lethal no matter when it is diagnosed. (Lerner 2000, 2001).
- Breast cancer is primarily genetic. Breast cancer is primarily environmental. (Rothman 1998; Steingraber 1998; Eisenstein 2001).
- Progress in medical research and practice has improved life expectancy for breast cancer patients (DeVita 1997). The mortality rate for breast cancer has changed little over the past century (Lerner 2001).
- The cure for breast cancer is within reach. Breast cancer is a collection of different diseases that take very different courses and will require different treatment strategies (Lerner 2001; Eisenstein 2001).
- All women are equally threatened by breast cancer. North American women contract breast cancer at higher rates than women in most other parts of the world and African-American women face exceptionally high mortality rates (Kasper and Ferguson 2000a; Shaffer 2000).
- All women over age 40 (or 50) should undergo annual mammograms. No woman should undergo routine mammograms (Weisman 2000).

3

M.C. Rawlinson and S. Lundeen (eds.), The Voice of Breast Cancer in Medicine and Bioethics, 3-19.
© 2006 *Springer. Printed in the Netherlands.*

- All women should practice regular breast self-examination. Regular breast self-examination may do more harm than good if widely practiced (Baxter 2001).
- Breast cancer begins in a specific location and spreads cells from that site in a gradual, orderly fashion to expanding circles of surrounding tissue; if caught early, it can be fully removed by excising all affected tissue.[1] Breast cancer is systemic; its cells spread through the body before any particular tumor can be located (Lerner 2001).
- The confusingly named "ductal carcinoma in situ" (DCIS) is a pre-curser to breast cancer that should be treated as if it were already breast cancer. DCIS is not cancer and in most cases it will not develop into cancer; it requires monitoring, not intervention (Zones 2000; Lerner 2001).
- Concerned individuals can best contribute to ending breast cancer by participating in national fund-raising efforts like the Pink Ribbon Campaign and the Race for the Cure. Concerned individuals should direct their energies and resources into supporting research programs designed to prevent breast cancer and lobbying for environmental changes (Batt 1994; Brenner 2000; Eisenstein 2001).
- Genetic testing holds promise of early detection and improved life expectancy for many women. At best, genetic tests can identify fewer than 10 percent of the women who will contract breast cancer in their lifetimes and it may not be able to save their lives (Rothman 1998).
- Women can protect themselves from breast cancer through conscientious compliance with expert medical advice, e.g., by engaging in healthful behaviors and watching for early signs of breast cancer. The only truly effective protection against breast cancer is social and environmental change through political action (Steingraber 2000; Eisenstein 2001).
- Tamoxifen and other drugs can reduce women's risks of contracting breast cancer and should be taken by all "high-risk" women. Until we have long-term data on the effectiveness and side effects of these drugs, women should view them as experimental interventions with their own associated risks (Batt 1994; Rosser 2000; Zones 2000).
- It is essential to promote hope among women diagnosed with breast cancer, so clinical settings should be cheerful and comforting places where patients are encouraged to look and feel feminine and attractive. Women diagnosed with breast cancer need access to clear, reliable, honest information; it should not be assumed that their primary concerns are with their appearance nor that they welcome being treated as children (Lorde 1980; Batt 1994; Ehrenreich 2001).

These are just a few of the many debates about breast cancer now raging around us. This paper is concerned with illuminating the problematic position that individual women encounter as they try to situate themselves within these debates. I am particularly interested in the difficulties faced by women who share feminism's appreciation of the political nature of many of these debates, but find themselves choosing personal strategies regarding breast cancer that may feel in tension with some of the political analyses they support. My aim is to show how the framing of breast cancer discourses shapes the decision-making of individual women and how that results in constraints on the ultimate autonomy of individual women in the realm of breast cancer. I shall also consider how women's autonomy might be expanded if we find ways of reformulating some of the discussions about breast cancer with alternative conceptions and images.

But first, two caveats. I shall not be offering any specific advice about the decisions particular women *should* make when confronting the threat or reality of breast cancer in their lives, nor will I be evaluating the quality of anyone's personal decision-making. Such judgments would, clearly, be an act of monumental hubris on my part. My focus is on the difficulties of the various choice situations women find themselves in when trying to protect themselves against the very real personal dangers posed by breast cancer.

Second, when I refer to the various perspectives in my title, I shall engage in some serious oversimplification. There are many different perspectives captured under each of the broad headings of "feminist," "medical," "scientific," and "commercial." Each of these categories comprises multiple positions representing significant differences of opinion.[2] Rather than engage directly in any of these internal debates, I shall focus only on some of the dominant views within each category. Moreover, I do not mean to imply that there is no space for people to hold multiple perspectives; in particular, I do not want to suggest that feminists never speak from a medical or scientific perspective, or, conversely, that it is impossible for scientists to adopt feminist insights and values. I shall use these four general categories as overlapping and interrelated positions, referring to some of the common assumptions that characterize each one, rather than to any essential beliefs of their various practitioners.

2. POLITICIZING THE PERSONAL

The best known, and probably the most important, message of the second wave of feminism is that the personal is political. This slogan emerged from the heady days of consciousness-raising activities in the 1960s and 1970s when women began to share stories of all aspects of their lives within loosely organized groups. They explored individual experiences in areas that had long been consigned to the realm of the personal and the private, with particular attention to sexual and reproductive experiences and desires; as they spoke about their intimate lives, they uncovered common patterns in the content and the contexts of their innermost thoughts and feelings. Once the patterns were identified, they could see how large social forces affected not only the public but also the personal spheres of their lives. With this recognition, it became possible to organize actions that would disrupt and, it was assumed, eventually end the pattern of male dominance in intimate relationships.

Thus, the slogan "the personal is political" reflects several major accomplishments. It captures the insight that what appears to be most personal and private often reflects and supports systemic power relationships between groups.

Specifically, the slogan illuminates patterns of domination that had long been ignored and it provides the grounds for challenging apparently "natural" gendered behaviors. It also empowers individual women to resist the specific enactments of those power relationships in their own lives. Consider gendered violence. Recognizing that the personal is political encourages women who have been victims of domestic or sexual violence to resist the tendency towards personal feelings of shame and failure and to develop instead a sense of righteous anger at the systemic extent of gender violence.

The slogan also makes clear that the required response to the problems revealed must be political (i.e., collective). In this function, it fits well with another important feminist slogan: there are no private solutions. That is, no woman can truly protect herself from gender violence within a world in which such violence is tolerated, even glamorized. This does not mean, however, that there is nothing that individual women can do: they can learn how to avoid particularly dangerous situations, defend themselves if attacked, and take retributive action against offenders. What they cannot do is to construct impenetrable defenses for themselves. True safety for individual women will only come when collective action succeeds in transforming the social conditions under which gendered violence thrives. Thus, feminists work politically to make social changes that will reduce the tendency of men to act violently and that will empower women and reduce their vulnerability to assault; in the present climate of continued gender violence, feminists also insist on appropriate services for those who suffer abuse.

3. POLITICIZING BREAST CANCER

Like matters of sexuality, domestic violence, and reproductive decision-making, breast cancer was long consigned to the domain of the private, even the secretive. Perhaps because there was a cloak of shame attached both to cancer and to the breast, most women with breast cancer were discouraged from discussing their condition in public (Rosenbaum and Roos 2000). Breast cancer emerged into the public domain in the 1970s, though in this case feminism was not the only force bringing it out into the open. The media took an active interest in the breast cancer experiences of such prominent women as Shirley Temple Black, Betty Ford, and Happy Rockefeller. These public figures graciously allowed their personal experiences to be used to help move breast cancer into public consciousness. Their rationale, presumably, was that such reports would encourage other women to check for early signs of tumors in the expectation that early detection supports early intervention and early intervention improves prognosis (Lerner 2001). In the subsequent decades, public discussion has increased steadily to the point that breast cancer is now a familiar topic of news reports and documentaries, the target of numerous advertising campaigns, and the focus of significant fund raising efforts. There is now an entire month devoted to breast cancer awareness.[3] As a result of all this attention, most Western women are not only aware of breast cancer, but tend to exaggerate their risk of contracting the disease (Kelly 1996).

Only certain dimensions of breast cancer are widely represented, however. Especially popular are the heroic tales of personal confrontations with breast cancer.[4] Generally, such stories are structured around an optimistic formula of hope and strength, though occasional reports of tragic outcomes serve as reminders that the battle is not yet won. The media also report on breast cancer fund-raising efforts, such as the annual Race for the Cure, and on government decisions to allocate money for research into breast cancer. Here, too, the message is strongly upbeat: resources are being directed at the search for a cure—which is portrayed as being just around the corner. In fact, casual readers and viewers of the news can be excused for thinking that the cure has already been found, since another popular news feature involves enthusiastic reports of scientific breakthroughs in the detection and successful treatment of breast cancer.[5]

Thus, frequent media reports, inspirational speakers, and plentiful self-help books and pamphlets have succeeded in removing breast cancer from the realm of the purely private and have made it a well known problem and subject of broad public concern. They stop far short of a feminist *politicizing* of the topic of breast cancer, however. Distinctively feminist analyses take a different form and end up with a different set of priorities regarding the disease. Many start in the same place, with a public discussion of a personal experience of breast cancer (e.g., Audre Lorde's *The Cancer Journals* and Sharon Batt's *Patient No More*), but feminist discussions go beyond reports of personal struggle to include reflection on how patterns of breast cancer incidence and dominant medical strategies relate to existing power structures.

Like feminism itself, feminist perspectives on breast cancer come in many different forms. In fact, they tend to reflect the many different approaches taken to feminism. The most visible and widely supported effort falls within the general framework of liberal feminism; this can be characterized as the movement to support patient choice over all aspects of her care. The need for individual control emerged as a high priority after women such as Babette Rosmond and Rose Kushner published personal accounts of their experiences with the disease.[6] These accounts differed dramatically from the more familiar stories in which doctors were typically portrayed as heroic rescuers. Rosmond, Kushner, and other women in this alternative genre challenged the routine medical care they were offered and reported on their struggles for personal control over treatment decisions (Lerner 2001). Their stories helped make public some of the intense medical debates about treatment options, revealing the disturbing fact that even the "experts" were not clear about the best course of action.

In the same time period, the courts and the newly evolved field of biomedical ethics exerted pressure on physicians to obtain fully informed consent from their patients before initiating treatments. These various forces helped to generate a widespread movement to a consumer model of medical interaction in which many patients came to insist on being informed and consulted about major medical interventions. Thus, through the 1970s and 1980s, many more women with breast cancer began to demand an active role in treatment decisions, such as the extent and timing of their surgeries. Often, patients demanded access to supplemental therapies such as chemotherapy and radiation; many even insisted on access to experimental treatments. As a result, feminists were able to make a strong case for empowering women as consumers of breast cancer care. Virtually all feminists were (and still are) determined to ensure that women understand the debates around mammography, mastectomies, chemotherapy, radiation, and other treatment options so that they can make informed, meaningful choices about their care. "Patient empowerment," understood as the opportunity to educate oneself on current medical thinking and to make one's own choice in the face of medical uncertainty, became a feminist slogan nearly everyone could support. It fits comfortably within the value system of a culture that prizes individual choice on matters of central importance in a person's life.

Not all feminists are satisfied with this solution, however, and many continue to struggle for a more comprehensive political analysis of breast cancer that encompasses a more radical set of demands. They brought to the realm of breast cancer the central feminist question of "Who benefits and who is harmed by the existing policies?" This led them to track the various interests at stake in mainstream research agendas and treatment protocols and to trace the political contours of the scientific and medical responses to breast cancer. This research has revealed the enormous profits being made in the realm of breast cancer. As Jane Zones observes, "cancer has many profit centers—detection, treatment, prevention, and even advocacy" (Zones 2000, 120). Moreover, she explains that in the cancer field, "it is often the scientists who are doing the selling" (ibid., 126) since the support of research programs and treatment centers constructed to address the epidemic of breast cancer constitute an economy dependent on continuing (and expanding) demand for services. This coincidence of interests among medical, scientific, and commercial practitioners has led many feminists to wonder about how women's well-being fits into the agendas of these powerful interest groups.

Here is a partial list of some of the major themes espoused by significant groups of feminists that are not captured by the liberal feminist demand for informed choice on the part of patients:

- The importance of understanding why the incidence of breast cancer has steadily increased in developed countries over the last century and what types of changes are required to reverse that pattern.
- Recognition of the ways in which breast cancer represents the hazards of industrialization inscribed on women's bodies.
- Consideration of the ways in which this disease interacts with cultural understandings about the breast.[7]
- The need for more research into breast health so that we can better situate our understanding of what goes wrong in breast cancer.
- Investigation of the ways in which differences among women associated with race, class, ethnicity and sexuality affect women's susceptibility to breast cancer and the prognosis of those who contract the disease.

- The urgent need for health reform to ensure that no women face financial, physical, or social barriers to adequate care.
- Pursuit of holistic treatment programs in which women are treated as adults in need of comprehensive, individualized care, where they are neither infantilized nor reduced to passive objects of technological interventions.

Most feminists insist that they will not be satisfied with a "cure" that involves significant risks, nor one that might help only a limited segment of the population affected by breast cancer. They seek a strategy of genuine prevention that will protect all women. Moreover, some feminists are skeptical of organizing around breast cancer at all. They are wary of a single-issue strategy that treats any particular disease as solvable apart from a broad women's health agenda (Weisman 2000).

4. RETURNING TO THE PERSONAL

In fact, so much feminist energy has gone into making the case that breast cancer is a political issue that I fear there is insufficient explicit feminist discussion of the fact that the equation goes both ways: not only is the personal political, but the political is still also personal. As Zillah Eisenstein observes:

> Bodies are always personal in that each of us lives in one in a particularly individual way. They are also political in that they have meanings that are more powerful than any of us can determine. Femaleness, color, beauty, health are carved on us without our choice…Breast cancer is one more challenge.[8] (Eisenstein 2001, 1)

While feminists must continue to act collectively to promote the agendas they have identified, every woman must make individual decisions about how she will respond to the risk or reality of breast cancer in her life. Few of the choices she faces are straightforward; most are the subject of contestation among experts with different orientations in this debate. Indeed, much excellent feminist work has documented just how unsatisfactory many of the current options are: how limited some are in their effectiveness (e.g., substituting early detection for true prevention), how costly many are to the overall well-being of many women (e.g., substituting one disease for another),[9] and how inaccessible many options are to all but the relatively affluent.

My question, then, is about the structure of the choice situations that women face. What are the forces that shape the options before each woman and how do these forces determine the weight assigned to various alternatives? My goal is to shed some light on some of the political dimensions that contribute to the structuring of the choice situation that confronts individual women concerned about breast cancer. By exploring ways in which various interests combine to influence women's sense of meaningful options, I hope to make clearer how feminism can help to promote a better array of options, each of which is supported by adequate information.

One more caveat: many of the options I mention as constituting women's choice situation are only available to women with very good health insurance and excellent medical care. Many, perhaps most, women actually have a far narrower set of options from which to choose (Kasper 2000; Shaffer 2000). Nothing in my discussion should be interpreted as providing moral justification for the existence of financial or social barriers to excellent health care services for all.

5. ABOUT LANGUAGE

One valuable tool for making visible the values and interests at play in the perspectives under review is to look closely at the language each uses to frame the subject of breast cancer and, thus, to position its own response to it. As Audre Lorde wisely noted, "it is necessary to scrutinize not only the truth of what we speak, but the truth of that language by which we speak it" (Lorde 1980, 22). Elsewhere, I have argued that it is important to pay attention to the choice of metaphors and images that are used to discuss important subjects (Sherwin 2001). Most of us were first taught the meaning of metaphors through poetry and we may be inclined to assume that metaphors are primarily decorative, providing colorful rhetorical flourishes to otherwise straightforward messages. Yet, metaphors carry with them far more than imaginative richness; they also transmit meaning and understanding. They are the principal tools available to explain abstract, problematic, or complex phenomena. They work by making analogies between the domain in need of explanation and another, usually more familiar, domain. Metaphors transfer the relationships that fit one field of activity into the other. For example, temperature relations—lukewarm, hot, sizzling, or cold—can be used to describe the current popularity of media stars or the success of athletes. When time is thought of as money, it makes sense to say it can be saved, invested, wasted, or generously shared. Metaphors are extremely important to our ability to make sense of the world. As Lakoff and Johnson have argued, "what we experience, and what we do every day is very much a matter of metaphor" (Lakoff and Johnson 1980, 3). Metaphors organize our thinking and they shape our experience.

As a result, metaphors structure the types of responses we are able to envision as appropriate to a particular domain. By determining our sense of possibilities, they shape our behavior. Thus, they have ethical significance. And because familiar metaphors are often implicit and unconscious, they may be read as simply descriptions of the phenomenon in question. They may become so commonplace that it is difficult even to imagine other ways of understanding the subject. Certainly, modern living makes it seem unquestionable that time really *is* money and should be treated by the same value calculations. To escape frenetic patterns of living in which we try to pack as many valued activities as possible into our days, making the best possible use of every moment, we may need to make a deliberate effort to think of time as something other than a precious, finite resource; we might, for example, try to think of it as a nurturing embrace to be enjoyed in the present, not always "banked" for the future. Thus, expanding the range of possible behaviors in a given domain may require transformation in the common metaphors used to discuss it. Because such transformations may require broad social change, and may, therefore, involve challenging existing power structures, metaphors also can have political significance.[10]

One of the ways of capturing feminist concerns about mainstream medical and scientific approaches to breast cancer is to reflect on two of the core metaphors that structure the approaches practitioners in these fields take when addressing the disease. Rather than look at each field in my title in isolation, I shall consider the implications of medicine, science, and commerce all sharing the same core metaphors to conceptualize and respond to breast cancer. Indeed, the problem that concerns me here is the way in which these three fields coalesce around one particular view of breast cancer. By mutually reinforcing one another's approaches, these three fields leave little space to identify and explore alternative conceptions of the disease; thus, they effectively exclude from serious consideration the possible strategies that might become visible under competing frameworks. My aim, then, is to explore how feminist understandings can be productively directed at resisting and countering these widely accepted formulations in ways that will expand women's ultimate autonomy.

The two metaphors I have in mind are the metaphor of breast cancer constructed as an enemy with whom we are at war and the related metaphor of each woman's body as the terrain on which the enemy advances. The warfare metaphor is dominant in nearly all discussions of breast cancer. It is so pervasive it is difficult even to recognize it as a metaphor, for surely breast cancer is an "enemy." It can be lethal and cause enormous suffering; we all want to destroy it. There are reasons to be wary, however, since references to a "war" on breast cancer encourage us to model our relationship and responses to breast cancer according to the types of behavior appropriate in war. Among other things, this implies that breast cancer is clearly an enemy, best approached through the coordinated efforts of a militaristic type of response. The language ensures high levels of fear about the disease and it implies that there is danger in assuming complacency in the face of this scourge. Modern war invites reliance on technological tools of surveillance and response designed to search and destroy enemy cells; side effects are accepted as the "collateral damage" to be expected in war.[11] Moreover, warfare is expensive; its very being justifies a major deployment of resources. It has an obvious urgency that takes priority over other social issues. In the area of health and health care, diseases worthy of being the targets of war are likely to receive more resources than other, more mundane forms of illness such as those associated with poverty and violence. And, of course, wars are best conducted along hierarchical lines of authority. Critical questioning is discouraged as it undermines morale and introduces confusion in the ranks.

Wars also require a battlefield; in this case, that battlefield is the bodies of women. Within the biomedical model shared by medicine, science, and industry, attention is focused on physiology and anatomy. The primary concern is to cure disease by manipulations at the cellular, hormonal, and genetic levels (Rosser 2000). In the case of breast cancer, anomalous cells are viewed as growing out of control, so the role of medical intervention is to eradicate these unruly cells and restore order. The woman who encompasses the body in question largely disappears from view as attention focuses on the proper weapons to attack the enemy lurking within.

Women, too, are expected to treat their bodies as battlefields wherein an all-out campaign may be necessary to eliminate the treacherous cells they harbor. They are assigned an important role to play in this fight, for they are responsible for the "first line of defense," and this involves participation in regular surveillance operations on their breasts (Lerner 2001, 59) and consent to whatever attacks medical experts judge necessary to destroy the enemy if it is detected. Even in the absence of any detectable breast cancer cells, women are taught to distrust their bodies as potential sites of betrayal.

Within this framework of danger, urgency, and fear, the personal strategies available to each woman to reduce her chances of dying of breast cancer involve medical interventions of various degrees of severity. Since many of these interventions are of some value to some women, and since scientists are still largely unable to predict which women will benefit from which treatment, the "safe" course is generally assumed to be the one of maximal intervention. The fact that each of these interventions—from the non-invasive breast self-examination and the painful mammography, through to surgery, chemotherapy, radiation, bone marrow transplants, and other experimental treatments—comes with costs and risks of its own seems irrelevant when the stakes are so high. When the battlefield is women's bodies, the war is fought in each body anew. Hence, as Maryann Napoli argues: "whether it is chemotherapy or radiotherapy, overtreatment of the majority to save a small minority has been the story of breast cancer treatment for decades" (Napoli 1999, 2). What may look like excessive risks and costs from an epidemiological perspective seems of unquestionable value from the personal perspective of each patient. In a war, individual survival is the highest priority.

The value of any metaphor lies in its ability to help us to understand a phenomenon better by analogy with some other domain. Particular metaphors may be so effective, though, that they actually mislead us. As analogies, metaphors are never perfect mirrors for the phenomenon in question. Moreover, metaphors are always contingent—they are approximations, not literal descriptions. Even as they illuminate certain dimensions of the phenomenon to which they are applied, they obscure other important aspects. There are always important differences between the two domains that may become difficult to detect when metaphors become entrenched. In fact, the more plausible the analogy, the more difficult it is to see its limitations.

The metaphors of breast cancer as an enemy with whom we are engaged in deadly warfare, fought on the bodies of women, support certain types of biomedical response to breast cancer. They make it very difficult, however, for us to see the possibilities of other ways of responding to breast cancer, other ways of defining the scope of the illness, or, especially, other ways of understanding the women who are diagnosed with the disease. Even if we cannot help but think of breast cancer as an enemy that threatens the lives of many women, there are many different ways of dealing with enemies other than open warfare.[12] As well, it is obvious that women are far more than geographical sites for breast cancer growth. It seems, however, that the urgency associated with the war imagery invoked in breast cancer "campaigns" makes attention to the complex experiences of women diagnosed with this disease far less important than the rapid deployment of technological weaponry.

It is clear that these metaphors serve the interests of medicine, science, and commerce well. They both motivate and justify the approaches to breast cancer taken by the majority of practitioners in all three domains, supporting their collaboration in a project that is seen by them and by the public to be very important, valuable work. Self-interest and public interest coincide seamlessly for people working in all three fields when breast cancer is understood according to the metaphors of war fought on the bodies of women. But feminists must ask how well these metaphors ultimately serve the interests of women.

6. UNDERSTANDING THE NATURE OF OUR CHOICES

My concern is that the metaphors of war and the associated sense of risk and danger leave no rational choice available to particular women but to participate fully in the regimes designed to fight the danger. When all three domains of science, medicine, and commerce appeal to the same metaphors and the same explanatory framework, their perspectives reinforce one another and make resistance seem unreasonable, dangerous, even foolish. As Barron Lerner observes, "it has become nearly impossible to discuss any initiative to prevent, detect, or treat breast cancer without using the language of battle" (Lerner 2001, 269). By sharing in this metaphorical depiction of the struggles associated with breast cancer, these three major areas of activity jointly seem to fill the available explanatory space and leave little room for exploration of alternative meanings or strategies.

Zillah Eisenstein observes:

> The cancer establishment's institutional base is located in the American Cancer Society, the National Cancer Institute, the Federal Drug Administration, the Environmental Protection Agency, the Department of Agriculture, and sectors of the American Medical Society. *Together* they network to articulate a cohesively authoritative breast cancer narrative. The cancer establishment favors cure over prevention, patentable and/or synthetic chemicals over natural and holistic methods. The contours and monies for research follow from this reference point…There is extraordinary interplay between the doctors who administer treatments, the scientists who do the research and set the trial, and the companies that sell the drugs. The FDA, NCI, and ACS all collaborate on treatments of choice, therapies, and diagnosis. (Eisenstein 2001, 101; emphasis added).

This powerful combination of authoritative voices structure public and private understandings and expectations of breast cancer. When individual women reflect on their own vulnerability to breast cancer and try to decide on the best strategy to reduce their own risk of dying of this disease, they must deliberate within the framework this coalition of forces has made available. This makes it very difficult to choose any but the dominant strategies in the various dualisms listed at the beginning of this paper. To refuse interventions developed within the dominant biomedical model in the face of a discourse of high risk and significant personal danger is widely viewed as irrational, even irresponsible, behavior.

Let me be very careful here. I am not claiming that it is *wrong* for women to choose any of the available medical treatments for preventing, detecting, or treating breast cancer. I, too, support the familiar liberal feminist agenda of empowering individual women to make the best choice they can by receiving full, accurate, and honest information about the options available to them; I, too, will insist that each woman have access to the treatments she prefers and not be deprived of good medical care by financial or social barriers. I am also not saying that physicians are wrong to offer women these options. At present, they seem to be important tools in any strategy to avoid the very real possibility of particular women dying of breast cancer; physicians are responsible for providing their patients with the option of treatments that have been proven effective.

What I am arguing is that the actual set of options each woman is "offered" contains only those interventions that have been generated within a research and practice agenda that has emerged from a particular understanding of the nature of breast cancer. The dominant model frames breast cancer as an enemy that must be attacked with all the weapons at our disposal. It makes it a moral duty of women to join the fight by delivering their bodies to medical authorities empowered to wield the high-tech interventions they have devised and to permit that fight to be pursued until either the woman or the cancer is destroyed. What is not available to women is a set of meaningful alternative ways to think about their own situation with respect to breast cancer and to respond in ways that address the threat that breast cancer poses to women collectively.

The options that emerge from the biomedical perspective built around these core metaphors depoliticize the context of the disease and encourage each woman to pursue an individualistic strategy built around a sense of high personal risk. This approach is analogous to trying to eradicate gender violence by offering every woman the opportunity to learn self-defense and improving the quality of emergency room care for victims of assault. These are important elements of a program to eliminate gender violence, but they are nowhere near sufficient to eradicate the problem. Similarly, as long as the focus remains on fighting breast cancer woman by woman, it is difficult to generate the political organization necessary to challenge the forces that may contribute to some instances of the disease by poisoning our environment, our food, or even the prescription drugs we take for other concerns (Steingraber 1998; Eisenstein 2001; Sharpe et al. 2002).

Under these circumstances, the best that individual women can achieve is a form of autonomy understood on the model of consumer choice, where one is free to choose among a finite number of pre-selected options. In the current climate, nearly all the medically authorized options have been developed within the same limited model of understanding breast cancer as a purely local, physiological phenomenon. In each case, the most rational choice tends to be pre-determined by the imagery of fighting the war on their bodies. Within this context, to refuse the biomedically approved protocol of the day seems to amount to irresponsible, premature surrender to a deadly force.

This type of informed choice within a narrow set of options should be seen as a limited form of autonomy. It accepts the choice situation as straightforward and evaluates the quality of the individual's decision-making capacity by judging her decisions as rational or not according to the information available to her. A richer conception, which I have called relational autonomy, requires us to evaluate not only the capacity of particular individuals to choose well under specific conditions, but also the circumstances in which individuals must make their choices.[13] Relational autonomy is "a capacity or skill that is developed (and constrained) by social circumstances. It is exercised within relationships and social structures that jointly help to shape the individual..." (Sherwin 1998, 36). Relational autonomy is sensitive to the ways in which power imbalances, especially those associated with oppression, can skew the array of choices available to support the interests of the powerful while constraining the capacity of the oppressed to find options that reduce their oppression.[14] We measure relational autonomy against the social and political conditions under which the choices in question are made.

Hence, when exploring the degree of relational autonomy that is present in a choice situation, it is necessary to consider whether adequate social conditions are in place to facilitate choices that support the interests of both the individual and whatever social groups she belongs to. As we have seen, most of the medical options available to individual women have been developed from within a common view of breast cancer built around the metaphors of warfare and risk factors. This limits women's relational autonomy in important ways. First, it means that the necessary research to support informed choices has been concentrated on one set of understandings of the disease. Possible research and treatment strategies that might emerge from other conceptions have simply not been pursued. Second, the options that have been developed all seem to fit within an approach to health and illness that concentrates power in the hands of medical and scientific experts and encourages dependence and deference on the part of frightened women.

To gain more autonomy, measured as a relational condition, we would need much more diversity in research approaches to breast cancer. We would need a research agenda that explores a range of different types of understandings and investigates different opportunities to alter the pattern of incidence. If research into breast cancer were pursued under this model, women's knowledge would not be limited to what commercially driven science has seen fit to study. It would also reflect the range of questions that feminists raise about breast cancer, including questions about how to promote breast health, the need to limit industrial activities that pose a risk to women's health (Rosser 2001), the reasons for racial and ethnic differences in diagnosis and mortality (Kasper and Ferguson 2000b), and the availability of strategies to live well despite the presence of breast cancer (Kasper and Ferguson 2000a).

The difficulties women face in making alternative understandings of breast cancer meaningful and vibrant are a result of the hegemony of the biomedical model. It is this hegemony that feminists challenge in their demands for genuine understanding and control over the disease in addition to adequate consumer-oriented responses in the absence of effective prevention strategies. So powerful is the coalition of voices working within the dominant biomedical model that it is difficult for anyone—patient, physician, or researcher—even to imagine alternative understandings of the disease.

Yet, it may be productive to think of breast cancer differently; for example, we might try to think of it as a potentially chronic condition. This framework would encourage us to view it not as an alien enemy but as a condition of life that should be addressed not by trying to eliminate all traces but through management of symptoms. The latter approach suggests adaptation to an intruder, perhaps even a destructive vandal, but not necessarily the annihilation of an invader whatever the cost. We might explore the metaphor of resilience to try to understand how we can help women who contract breast cancer to avoid its potentially deadly impact. Under such metaphors, we might look for "civil" strategies to promote the well-being of the "community," but we would be less inclined to focus on missions of sheer destruction. These alternative metaphors may generate a more appropriate understanding for women whose breast cancer cannot be cured and who must come to terms with living out their lives in the presence of the disease. They also capture the fact that some forms of breast cancer appear to be very slow growing and may be present in women's bodies for decades without causing them serious illness.

Feminism does not provide prescriptive advice to women struggling to decide their own strategies around breast cancer any more than it can tell particular women how to conduct their lives in the face of ongoing threats of gender violence. What it can and does do is to make clear why an array of "choices" from within a single narrow framework limits the genuine autonomy of individual women and undermines the interests of women collectively. In breast cancer as in gender violence, it seems likely that threats to individual well-being can only be fully addressed by broad social changes achieved through political action. In the meantime, feminism can help us to understand that adequate personal strategies require having available meaningful and satisfactory choices. In order to develop the range of options required by a feminist agenda for breast cancer, it will be necessary to supplement the dominant framework by developing alternative ways of thinking about health and disease in general, and, particularly, about breast health and breast disease.

Susan Sherwin, Ph.D., FRSC, is a University Research Professor of Philosophy and Women's Studies at Dalhousie University with a cross appointment to the Department of Bioethics.

NOTES

I wish to thank the many readers and listeners who took the time and interest to engage with the ideas in this paper at Stony Brook University, Dalhousie University, and Memorial University. I am particularly grateful to Sharon Batt, Françoise Baylis, Richmond Campbell, Sue Campbell, Carmel Forde, and Michael Hymers for their insightful contributions and Thane Plantikow for her conscientious assistance.

1. Lerner (2000, 2001) documents this as the dominant understanding that supported the use of the Halsted radical mastectomy for many years.

2. In fact, some of the differences of opinion within science and medicine are so extreme they have been described in the language of war, as in the provocative titles of Barron Lerner's book *The Breast Cancer Wars* (2001) and Robert Proctor's *Cancer Wars* (1995).

3. It is worth noting that the principal sponsor of Breast Cancer Awareness Month (BCAM) is AstraZeneca, the company that produces and markets Tamoxifen. It retains authority to approve or disapprove all printed material used in BCAM (Zones 2000).

4. These narratives make compelling stories and they serve multiple purposes. They serve as cautionary tales, warning other women of the ever-present threat of breast cancer and thus encouraging them to participate in screening programs to facilitate early detection and, thereby, early interventions. They also encourage support for fund-raising efforts and research programs aimed at a cure. And, typically, these personal stories provide role models of particular women's courage in the face of a serious health crisis, reminding everyone that there is life after a diagnosis of breast cancer and that it is a battle worth fighting. Particularly popular are stories in which a diagnosis of breast cancer helps a woman to find meaning in her life and represents an opportunity for personal growth.

5. Not infrequently, these reports describe some discovery so exciting the scientists cannot even wait to complete their testing protocols before going public with their "very promising results" (e.g., the initial trial with Tamoxifen as a preventive measure for healthy women who are deemed to be at high risk of contracting breast cancer). Typically, scientific breakthroughs are reported with scant reference to potential problems or limits to the new intervention.

6. For more discussion of Kushner and Rosmond's activism, see Barron Lerner's chapter in this volume. See also, Kushner (1975).

7. For example, how do we understand the cultural expectations of women's bodies when medicine is preoccupied with removal of diseased (or potentially diseased) breasts, and at the same time is committed to offering women reconstructive surgery and is engaged in the widespread surgery of breast augmentation on healthy breasts?

8. I note that Zillah Eisenstein (2001) has also found the metaphors of politicizing the personal and personalizing the political a helpful way to organize her discussion of breast cancer from a personal and political perspective. Her first chapter is titled "Personalizing the Political" and her second "Politicizing the Personal." I chose my title for this paper independently but I have found her book immensely valuable in organizing my own thinking on the subject.

9. The high rate of complications associated with administering Tamoxifen as a preventative measure to women who have not been diagnosed with breast cancer is often described by critics as substituting one disease (endometrial cancer) for another (breast cancer).

10. In Sherwin (2001), I argued that this is the situation with regard to the metaphors used to refer to HIV/AIDS and the policies aimed at controlling its spread and effects.

11. In fact, most of the tools deployed against breast cancer emerge from the same technology as the production of weapons for war, establishing that even weapons of destruction can have positive social value and providing additional support for investments in this sort of technology.

12. Even within the war metaphor, we may need to be more sophisticated about our understanding of the type of war we are engaged in. Is it a conventional war, an all-out nuclear war, or a new-style war on terrorism? Different strategies attach to different types of wars.

13. See my essay, "A relational approach to autonomy in health care," (Sherwin 1998).

14. Frye proposes that the double bind—in which there is no non-oppressive option—is a defining condition of oppression (Frye 1983, 2).

REFERENCES

Batt, Sharon. 1994. *Patient No More: The Politics of Breast Cancer*. Charlottetown: Gynergy Books.

Baxter, Nancy with the Canadian Task Force on Preventive Health Care. 2001. Preventive health care, 2001 update: Should women be routinely taught breast self-examination to screen for breast cancer? *Canadian Medical Association Journal* 164, no. 13 (June 26): 1837-46.

Brenner, Barbara A. Sister support: Women create a breast cancer movement. In *Breast Cancer: Society Shapes an Epidemic*, ed. Anne S. Kasper and Susan J. Ferguson, 325-353. New York: St. Martin's Press.

DeVita, Vincent T., Jr. 1997. The war on cancer has a birthday and a present. *Journal of Clinical Oncology* 15: 867-869.

Ehrenreich, Barbara. 2001. Welcome to cancerland: A mammogram leads to a culture of pink kitsch. *Harpers*, November: 43-53.

Eisenstein, Zillah. 2001. *Manmade Breast Cancers*. Ithaca: Cornell University Press.

Foskat, Jennifer R., Angela Karran, and Christine LaFia. 2000. Breast cancer in popular women's magazines from 1913-1996. In *Breast Cancer: Society Shapes an Epidemic*, ed. Anne S. Kasper and Susan J. Ferguson, 303-323. New York: St. Martin's Press.

Frye, Marilyn. 1983. *The Politics of Reality: Essays in Feminist Theory*. Freedom, CA: Crossing Press.

Kasper, Anne S. 2000. Barriers and burdens: Poor women face breast cancer. In *Breast Cancer: Society Shapes an Epidemic*, ed. Anne S. Kasper and Susan J. Ferguson, 183-212. New York: St. Martin's Press.

Kasper, Anne S. and Susan J. Ferguson. 2000a. Conclusion: Eliminating breast cancer from our future. In *Breast Cancer: Society Shapes an Epidemic*, ed. Anne S. Kasper and Susan J. Ferguson, 355-373. New York: St. Martin's Press.

Kasper, Anne S. and Susan J. Ferguson. 2000b. Living with breast cancer. In *Breast Cancer: Society Shapes an Epidemic*, ed. Anne S. Kasper and Susan J. Ferguson, 1-22. New York: St. Martin's Press.

Kelly, Patricia T. 1996. Cancer risk information services: Promise and pitfalls. *Breast Journal* 2: 233-37.

Kushner, R. 1975. *Breast Cancer: A Personal and an Investigative Report*. New York: Harcourt Brace Jovanovich.

Lakoff, George and Mark Johnson. 1980. *Metaphors We Live By.* Chicago: University of Chicago Press.

Lerner, Barron H. 2001. *The Breast Cancer Wars: Hope, Fear, and the Pursuit of a Cure in Twentieth-Century America.* Oxford: Oxford University Press.

——— 2000. Inventing a curable disease: Historical perspectives on breast cancer. In *Breast Cancer: Society Shapes an Epidemic*, ed. Anne S. Kasper and Susan J. Ferguson, 25-49. New York: St. Martin's Press.

Lorde, Audre. 1980. *The Cancer Journals.* San Francisco: Spinsters/Aunt Lute.

Napoli, Maryann. 1999. Breast removal: The latest in cancer prevention. *HealthFacts*, February: 1-2.

Proctor, Robert. 1995. *Cancer Wars: How Politics Shapes What We Know and Don't Know About Cancer.* New York: Basic Books.

Rosenbaum, Marcy E. and Gun M. Roos. 2000. Women's experiences of breast cancer. In *Breast Cancer: Society Shapes an Epidemic*, ed. Anne S. Kasper and Susan J. Ferguson, 153-181. New York: St. Martin's Press.

Rosser, Sue V. 2000. Controversies in breast cancer research. In *Breast Cancer: Society Shapes an Epidemic*, ed. Anne S. Kasper and Susan J. Ferguson, 245-270. New York: St. Martin's Press.

Rothman, Barbara Katz. 1998. *Genetic Maps and Human Imaginations: The Limits of Science in Understanding Who We Are.* New York: W.W. Norton & Company, Inc.

Shaffer, Ellen R. 2000. Breast cancer and the evolving health care system: Why health care reform is a breast cancer issue. In *Breast Cancer: Society Shapes an Epidemic*, ed. Anne S. Kasper and Susan J. Ferguson, 89-118. New York: St. Martin's Press.

Sharpe, C.R., J.P. Collet, E. Belzile, J.A. Hanley, and J.F. Biovin. 2002. The effects of tricyclic antidepressants on breast cancer risk. *British Journal of Cancer* 86, no. 1 (January, 7): 92-97.

Sherwin, Susan. 2001. Feminist ethics and the metaphors of AIDS. *Journal of Medicine and Philosophy* 26, no. 4: 343-364.

——— 1998. A relational approach to autonomy in health care. In The Feminist Health Care Ethics Research Network, Susan Sherwin Co-ordinator, *The Politics of Women's Health: Exploring Agency and Autonomy*, 19-47. Philadelphia: Temple University Press.

Steingraber, Sandra. 1998. *Living Downstream: A Scientist's Personal Investigation of Cancer and the Environment.* New York: Vintage Books.

Weisman, Carol S. 2000. Breast cancer policymaking. In *Breast Cancer: Society Shapes an Epidemic*, ed. Anne S. Kasper and Susan J. Ferguson, 213-243. New York: St. Martin's Press.

Zones, Jane A. 2000. Profits from pain: The political economy of breast cancer. In *Breast Cancer: Society Shapes an Epidemic*, ed. Anne S. Kasper and Susan J. Ferguson, 119-151. New York: St. Martin's Press.

CHAPTER TWO

BARRON H. LERNER, M.D., Ph.D.

POWER, GENDER, AND PIZZAZZ

The Early Years of Breast Cancer Activism

"Now the surgeon is faced with a patient," wrote an alarmed breast cancer physician in 1974, "who presents herself with a lump in her breast, a copy of an article from *Vogue* magazine, a quotation from the *Today* show, and a preconceived notion of how she should be treated" (Wilson 1974, 407). Today, clinicians fully expect breast cancer patients to get second opinions, search the Internet, and read articles about the disease in women's magazines and on the Internet. But it was less than thirty years ago that such behavior was unexpected and even resented. How did such a change occur?

This paper will examine the rise of modern breast cancer activism in the 1970s. In this decade, large numbers of women challenged the authority of the medical profession for the first time. Their efforts were intimately related to feminism, reflecting a larger call for women's rights throughout American society. At the same time, these attempts to change medical practice were tied to the rise of a new consumerist ethos.

By the end of the 1970s, breast cancer patients had helped to transform the ways in which treatment decisions were made for all diseases. In addition, they helped make breast cancer a compelling health issue for Americans, a process that would accelerate in subsequent decades. Yet despite achieving numerous successes, the breast cancer activists of the 1970s unearthed a series of complicated problems that remain unresolved today.

THE WAY IT WAS

To understand what breast cancer activists achieved in the 1970s, it is first necessary to understand how doctors and patients interacted prior to this decade. In this era,

M.C. Rawlinson and S. Lundeen (eds.), The Voice of Breast Cancer in Medicine and Bioethics, 21-30.

physicians largely called the shots. Doctors did not offer patients treatments for various diseases. Rather, they told women which therapy they would receive.

Physician authority was especially notable in the case of breast cancer (Lerner 2001, 15-40). In the late nineteenth century, famed Johns Hopkins University surgeon, William S. Halsted, had popularized an operation known as the radical mastectomy. Women who underwent this dramatic operation lost not only the cancerous breast and nearby lymph nodes, but also both chest wall muscles on the side of the cancer. Embodying the possibilities of scientific medicine and the power of the American surgical profession, the radical mastectomy vanquished less disfiguring treatment options being used in Canada and Europe.

Building on the Allied victory in World War II, the surgical "war" on breast cancer accelerated after 1945. Surgeons at New York's Memorial Sloan-Kettering Cancer Center and the University of Minnesota pioneered the extended radical mastectomy, which involved removing portions of the rib cage in search of elusive cancer cells. In retrospect, the use of such disfiguring operations accelerated because surgeons conflated their efforts in the operating room with actual clinical outcomes (Lerner 2001, 69-91). However, women at the time, believing that such aggressive surgery improved their chances of cure, readily, if regretfully, submitted to such procedures. For example, when Marion Flexner's physician-husband informed her that she would need radical surgery if her breast lump proved cancerous, Flexner "tried hard not to disappoint him" (Flexner 1947, 57).

The degree to which physicians controlled decision-making regarding breast and other cancers in the 1950s and 1960s is underscored by their routine concealment of the diagnosis from victims of the disease. Up to 90 percent of doctors, generally with the family's approval, preferred not to tell patients–women and men–that they had cancer (Oken 1961). Euphemisms such as "tumor" or "growth" were used instead. Obviously, such uninformed persons could not participate meaningfully in any treatment decisions. It is true that certain breast cancer patients declined radical surgery, instead requesting a less extensive operation or radiotherapy. But such cases proved to be the exception.

By the late 1960s, numerous groups in American society, ranging from civil rights activists to anti-Vietnam War demonstrators, were challenging authority. Medicine, which had experienced a golden era following the successful development of penicillin and the polio vaccine, was itself under siege. The Tuskegee scandal, in which poor African American men with syphilis were left untreated for research purposes, hit the newspapers in 1972 (Jones 1993). Concurrently, it was learned that investigators had intentionally infected retarded children with the hepatitis virus at a New York institution named Willowbrook (Rothman and Rothman 1984). Physicians, it appeared, were as likely as other establishment groups in society to exploit those less powerful.

Meanwhile, feminists argued that sexism was rampant in the United States. Men, they claimed, both discriminated against women and treated them in a condescending manner. Such concerns quickly spread to health care, where women activists began to criticize what they believed was the unequal relationship between doctors and patients, particularly surrounding issues of contraception and childbirth (Seaman 1969; Ruzek 1978). The need for women to question their obstetricians received extensive attention in the first edition of *Our Bodies, Ourselves*, a health manual published in 1970 by what became known as the Boston Women's Health Book Collective.

The women who became breast cancer activists did not act on their own. Rather, they incorporated the arguments of a small group of iconoclastic physicians who had been questioning medicine's unwavering allegiance to radical surgery for over a dozen years. One was Oliver Cope of Boston's Massachusetts General Hospital. In 1970, Maryel Locke, the editor of the *Radcliffe Quarterly*, convinced Cope to write an article, "Breast Cancer: Has the Time Come for a Less Mutilating Treatment?" (Cope 1970). The piece was quickly reprinted in Vogue. Meanwhile, George (Barney) Crile, Jr., of the Cleveland Clinic was writing a book, *What Women Should Know About the Breast Cancer Controversy* (Crile 1973). Both men argued that radical mastectomies made no sense. For women with early cancer localized to the breast, they were too extensive; for those with advanced cancer, they were too late. Despite some supportive data, Cope's and Crile's calls for less radical surgery had largely fallen on deaf ears. But as breast cancer patients began to demand participation in their medical care, the words of these renegade surgeons would serve as an inspiration.

WOMEN IN REVOLT

Among the first such women was Babette Rosmond. Rosmond was a fifty-year-old fiction editor and writer at *Seventeen* magazine when she discovered a breast lump in February 1971. By the time she consulted a breast surgeon, Rosmond already had considered her options if the lump turned out to be cancerous. Two of her friends had experienced bad side effects following radical mastectomy. One still cried about having lost both her breast and chest wall muscles. The other had an extremely swollen arm and excruciating pain where the muscles had been removed. "The nerves in the stump of the pectoral muscle," she told Rosmond, "are screaming" (Lerner 2001, 152). Once Rosmond learned that certain doctors were questioning radical surgery, she had no intention of following in her friends' footsteps.

Rosmond was well-suited to challenge the medical profession. In contrast to most women of her generation, she worked full-time and had declined to take her husband's name. Although she disliked the term "feminist," she most certainly behaved like one. When a biopsy of Rosmond's lump came back as a tiny eight-millimeter cancer, her surgeon informed her that she needed an immediate radical mastectomy. Rosmond said no. Like most physicians of the era, Rosmond's surgeon was entirely unaccustomed to this type of challenge. He responded by invoking his professional authority, terming Rosmond "a very silly and stubborn woman." When she requested three weeks before making her final decision, the surgeon turned grim. "In three weeks," he announced with great hyperbole, "you may be dead" (Campion 1972, 33, 45).

It was not only breast surgeons who recoiled at the actions of patients such as Rosmond. Beginning in the 1960s, a series of psychiatrists and psychologists had begun to study the emotional repercussions of radical breast surgery. Although very sympathetic to the plight of such women, these researchers nevertheless viewed breast cancer patients who pursued alternative surgical options as crazy. Questioning one's physician, evidently, was pathological behavior.

Rosmond eventually made her way to the Cleveland Clinic, where she met with Barney Crile. As expected, Crile provided Rosmond with a series of choices, one of which was a partial mastectomy entailing removal of the cancer with preservation of the breast. (Today this operation is known as a lumpectomy.) Noting the small size of her cancer and that there was no evidence of spread, Rosmond chose this option. She also declined radiotherapy to the breast and underarm, which was generally given to patients who chose such limited surgery.

In 1972, using the pseudonym Rosamond Campion, Rosmond went public. She published an article about her experiences in *McCall's* magazine, entitled "The Right to Choose," and then expanded it into a book, *The Invisible Worm* (Campion 1972). Rosmond's words underscored her message. "I alone am in charge of my body," she stated. Reflecting on how she had stood up to her physicians, she wrote, "I think what I did was the highest level of women's liberation. I said 'No' to a group of doctors who told me 'You must sign this paper, you don't have to know what it's all about'" (Klemesrud 1972, 56). Central to Rosmond's credo was the importance of finding physicians who would listen to and respect their patients.

Rosmond's writings briefly made her a media celebrity. She appeared on the *Today* and *David Susskind* shows, where she debated a series of physicians. More bemused than angry, the petite Rosmond interrupted and challenged these doctors, even criticizing statements made by her physician, Crile. Although she carefully emphasized that her choice of partial mastectomy was a personal one, and that she was not recommending it for other women, her brash attitude exasperated her fellow guests. "The worst doctor is his own doctor," warned one physician. Another cautioned that women should not participate in decisions "so professional, so technical, so involved, so biological that they cannot begin to understand the facts" (Lerner 2001, 166). At one point, Susskind even called Rosmond "Mrs. Civilian," seemingly to remind her that she was not a physician.

The traditional roles of doctor and patient became further blurred thanks to another breast cancer activist, Rose Kushner. Kushner, a Washington, D.C. journalist who had covered medical, political and military topics, discovered a breast "elevation" in June 1974. Nineteen-seventy four would prove to be a crucial year in the history of breast cancer activism. In the fall of that year, both First Lady Betty Ford and Happy Rockefeller, wife of Vice President-elect Nelson Rockefeller, were diagnosed with the disease. The candor of these women made breast cancer, formerly cloaked in secrecy, a household term.

Upon detecting the abnormality in her breast, Kushner first proceeded not to a doctor but to the National Library of Medicine where she discovered Crile's book. Through her research, Kushner learned not only that certain physicians were questioning the radical mastectomy, but that the decision to proceed with this operation was generally made while a woman was under anesthesia. That is, an intraoperative biopsy showing breast cancer became an indication for immediate radical surgery. To Kushner, this "one-step" procedure silenced a woman during one of the most important moments of her life.

Kushner had great difficulty finding a surgeon who would perform a two-step operation, which would allow her to evaluate treatment options upon learning her diagnosis. Finally, she convinced her family surgeon to perform only a breast biopsy. When the result came back as positive, he could not contain his anger at having performed an unorthodox procedure. Rattling the bars of Kushner's hospital bed, he snapped, "I never should have let you get away with it!" (Robertson 1979, 6). Having learned she had cancer, Kushner next struggled to find a surgeon willing to perform a so-called modified radical mastectomy, which removed the breast but left the chest wall muscles in place.

Kushner was not one to let such outrageous experiences go unreported. Possessed of, by her own admission, "a streak of stubbornness and a loud voice," she embarked on "a crusade to tell American women—and through them American doctors—what I have learned." "Vietnam," she announced in typical fashion, "would have to wait" (Lerner 2001, 177). Kushner quickly placed an article in the *Washington Post* and then published a book, *Breast Cancer: A Personal and Investigative History*, in 1975 (Kushner 1975).

In contrast to Rosmond, Kushner made breast cancer the subsequent focus of her professional life. Capitalizing on the new attention being given to the disease, Kushner appeared across the country, urging breast cancer patients to become active in making medical decisions. She also began the Breast Cancer Advisory Center, which provided advice by mail and phone to thousands of women confronting a diagnosis of breast cancer. Kushner's efforts inspired other activists to form self-help groups, such as SHARE and Y-ME, for women with breast and other cancers.

In her early years as a breast cancer activist, Kushner was extremely confrontational. As a journalist, she gained admission to medical meetings, where she used her articulateness and humor to disrupt the proceedings. Most importantly, she ably challenged the data that doctors were presenting. As was the case with Rosmond, many physicians responded defensively when Kushner–a lay woman– questioned their authority. One doctor termed her book "a piece of garbage" (Robertson 1979, 6).

Kushner's targets were not limited to the medical profession. Upon learning in October 1974 that First Lady Betty Ford would have a one-step radical mastectomy should her biopsy show cancer, she phoned the White House to object. She was rebuffed, being told by her friend and presidential advisor Milton Friedman that, "The President has made his decision." Infuriated by this "male-chauvinist piggery," Kushner later wrote, "[t]hat line has got to be engraved somewhere as the all-time sexist declaration of no-woman rights" (Lerner 2001, 179).

Kushner experienced her greatest triumph at a 1979 National Institutes of Health conference on the treatment of breast cancer. Reflecting her remarkable knowledge of the disease, she had been chosen as the only lay member of the consensus panel. Not only did the panel declare the radical mastectomy obsolete, something that Kushner had been advocating for five years, but it also included a statement rejecting the one-step approach to breast cancer diagnosis and treatment. Women would no longer be the silent partner in the doctor-patient relationship.

VANITY AND APPEARANCE

Once activists like Rosmond and Kushner had made it acceptable for women to assert their rights, other breast cancer patients began to speak out on related topics. One major concern was the emotional impact of breast cancer, both at the time of diagnosis and when a woman underwent disfiguring surgery as part of her treatment. Betty Rollin, who was diagnosed with breast cancer in 1975, candidly addressed this issue.

By entitling her 1976 account of her experiences *First, You Cry*, Rollin emphasized that crying was an appropriate response to the diagnosis of breast cancer. Moreover, Rollin's book openly discussed a series of controversial topics—appearance, vanity and sexuality. Even though most patients suffered fewer side effects than had Rosmond's friends, all women who underwent radical mastectomy were left with a sunken, scarred chest wall and difficulty wearing low-cut dresses. For Rollin, a television correspondent for NBC News, such an outcome was distressing. "I am vain," she told her surgeon prior to her modified radical mastectomy. "I would like to not be very hideous if that's possible" (Rollin 1976a, 58).

After the surgery, Rollin dealt openly with the grieving process that may accompany loss of a breast. When she first looked at her mastectomy scar, she informed readers, she felt "ugly and freaky; that anybody who saw me would be repelled and revolted the way I had been" (Rollin 1976b, 149). Rollin also frankly discussed her sex life in the months following her operation. In the process of divorcing her husband, she began an affair with another man who had dealt with her disease maturely and compassionately.

Perhaps even more than the writings of Rosmond and Kushner, Rollin's words cut against the grain. When confronted with a lethal disease like breast cancer, women were expected to be soldiers, maintaining a stiff upper lip. Loss of a breast, in other words, was the price one had to pay for the possibility of survival. Many physicians were appalled by women willing to ponder their looks in the face of breast cancer. Avoidance of adequate surgery due to "feminine whims," warned one, might result in a "dead woman with a somewhat more pleasant-appearing chest wall" (Ariel 1978, 62). Another doctor crudely opined that a breast cancer patient just needed to stuff an old stocking in her bra and get on with her life.

Not surprisingly, many women responded very positively to Rollin's candor. One woman remarked that she had finally read about another breast cancer patient "who had the same crazys [sic] I had." Another admitted that she, too, had stood in front of her mirror and said, "You ugly thing." A seventy-seven-year-old woman who had undergone a mastectomy told Rollin: "You would think that I wouldn't be so vain! But that's the way it is" (Lerner 2001, 185).

Interestingly, over time, Rollin came to downplay her earlier concerns about the effects of breast cancer and its treatment on her appearance. In 1980, for example, she chided herself for having been so fixated on wearing strapless dresses after her surgery. "Losing a breast is not so bad," Rollin later wrote. "It only seemed so at the time" (Rollin 1980, 37). Indeed, she had already begun to consider this perspective at the end of *First, You Cry*. Coining a memorable phrase, that surgery had left her with a "dent in my fender," she nevertheless noted that she was the same car that she had always been (Rollin 1976a, 230).

This notion—that one's life could largely return to normal after breast cancer— rankled Audre Lorde. Lorde, an African American writer and professor of English in New York City, developed breast cancer in 1978. In publicizing her experiences with the disease in *The Cancer Journals*, Lorde's message was novel. While she respected the efforts of earlier activists, she noted that women like Ford and Rollin had little to say to African American women with breast cancer. Lorde recounted how, after her mastectomy, she had been given a white lambswool breast form that looked "grotesquely pale" compared with her black skin (Lorde 1980, 44). Nor did existing breast cancer activism address the concerns of another group to which Lorde belonged—lesbians. She wrote that as a black, lesbian feminist poet, she had no role models.

It was Lorde's feminism that led her to reject the idea that her life would ever return to normal. "And yet if I cried for a hundred years," she wrote about her mastectomy, "I couldn't possibly express the sorrow I feel right now, the sadness and the loss" (Lorde 1980, 35). Lorde responded with particular antagonism toward the growing use of reconstructive breast surgery to restore a woman's preoperative appearance. On a practical level, she feared that such prostheses would potentially interfere with the detection of future cancers. But it was another type of concealment that bothered her even more. By undergoing reconstruction, a woman was attempting to erase a profound event—breast cancer—from her life. It was much more important, Lorde argued, for a breast cancer patient to continually reflect on her experiences, which would enable her to live a more considered, thoughtful life. One woman who embodied Lorde's philosophy was Deena Metzger, a spiritual healer who proudly displayed her mastectomy scar in her famous 1979 "warrior" poster (Lerner 2001, 270).

Beyond Lorde's concern that reconstruction rendered breast cancer invisible, she also questioned the motivations of male doctors who advocated reconstruction. Plastic surgeons, she wrote, were "sexist pigs" who exploited breast cancer patients and "remade their bodies into a configuration pleasing to the male eye" (Lorde 1980, 69).

CONCLUSION

What happened to these four women activists and the beliefs that they espoused? Babette Rosmond survived her breast cancer, dying in 1997, 26 years after her diagnosis. Interestingly, she probably died of a new breast cancer. A few years before her death, Rosmond had felt another lump. However, beginning to lose her memory, she decided not to have a biopsy. She gradually became more ill and likely died of metastatic cancer. Rosmond had made her own choice once again.

Rosmond lived to see scientific confirmation of her initial hunch about the treatment of localized breast cancer. Studies published in the 1980s by Bernard Fisher and others demonstrated that lumpectomies were as effective as any type of mastectomy–either radical or less extensive (Lerner 2001, 226). Rosmond also saw women gain the "right to choose" that she had so ardently promoted. Modern breast cancer patients who consult multiple physicians are no longer derided as "shopping" for second opinions but are respected as wise consumers.

Rose Kushner died of metastatic breast cancer in 1990, 16 years after her initial diagnosis. Between 1974 and her death, she remained America's most prominent breast cancer activist. Yet over time, Kushner became more of an insider than an outsider, lobbying for research funding and urging states across the country to pass informed consent laws for breast cancer treatment. In 1980 President Jimmy Carter selected her as the first lay member of the National Cancer Advisory Board. Having helped win women the right to make treatment decisions, Kushner increasingly stressed the importance of good science. She became a strong advocate of randomized controlled trials as the best mechanism for determining diagnostic and treatment strategies for breast cancer (Lerner 2001, 227-229). Seen from this perspective, Kushner was as much a consumer advocate as feminist critic of the system.

In 1991, with the formation of the National Breast Cancer Coalition, Kushner's lone wolf activism had matured into a highly professionalized advocacy movement (Belkin 1996). Thanks largely to the National Breast Cancer Coalition (NBCC), federal funding for breast cancer over the last decade has increased sevenfold to over $700 million annually. This money, plus funding from private organizations such as the Avon Corporation and the Susan Komen Foundation, has supported basic research into successful new interventions, such as the medication Herceptin.

Yet despite these achievements, critics have questioned aspects of modern breast cancer activism, most notably its focus on early detection and aggressive chemotherapy as opposed to prevention of the disease (Lerner 2002). The movement, it is argued, has paid insufficient attention to toxic waste and other possible environmental causes of breast cancer. Having drifted too far from its grassroots origins and too close to corporate America, breast cancer activism has become "a growth industry in a capitalist marketplace" (Kasper and Ferguson 2000, 358). It is interesting to speculate how Kushner would have responded to these critiques. Given her inherent distrust of complacency, she would likely have welcomed these newer attempts to think "outside the box."

Betty Rollin remains a correspondent for NBC News. After developing cancer in her second breast in 1984, she underwent another mastectomy followed by bilateral reconstruction. In a recent 25th anniversary edition of *First, You Cry*, Rollin approvingly likened her reconstructed breasts to "little waterbeds" that "stay up by themselves" (Rollin 2001, 219). Her once controversial concerns about the physical and emotional effects of breast cancer have gone mainstream, perhaps best exemplified by the American Cancer Society's "Look Good...Feel Better" program, which sees improved appearance as an important strategy for enhancing psychological recovery (Lerner and Rollin 2001). Meanwhile, breast reconstruction has become the norm for women who undergo mastectomies.

In this sense, most women have rejected Audre Lorde's attack on the procedure as sexist. Yet another goal emphasized by Lorde, who died of breast cancer in 1992, has become central to modern control efforts: studying how the disease impacts African Americans, lesbians and other often-neglected populations. Over the last decade, Congress has funded programs that fund free screening of poor women for cervical and breast cancer. Funding is also available to pay for treatment of those diagnosed with either disease.

Finally, Lorde's question about whether breast cancer patients can ever return to normal lives remains as provocative as ever. While some survivors prominently participate in walks, runs, mountain climbs and even parachute jumps "for the cure," other women quietly attempt to put their disease behind them. As the pioneer activists of the 1970s remind us, we should celebrate the diversity of choices made by breast cancer patients.

Dr. Lerner is Angelica Berrie-Gold Foundation Associate Professor of Medicine and Public Health at Columbia University. Funding for Dr. Lerner's research came from the Greenwall Foundation, the National Library of Medicine, and the Robert Wood Johnson Generalist Faculty Physician Scholar Program.

REFERENCES

Ariel, I.M. 1978. The treatment of breast cancer by radical and super radical mastectomy. *Resident & Staff Physician* (September): 57-62.

Belkin, L. 1996. How breast cancer became this year's hot charity. *New York Times Magazine*, December, 26: 40-57.

Campion, R. 1972. *The Invisible Worm: A Woman's Right to Choose an Alternate to Radical Surgery*. New York: Macmillan.

Cope, O. 1970. Breast cancer: Has the time come for a less mutilating treatment? *Radcliffe Quarterly*, June: 6-11.

Crile, G. 1973. *What Women Should Know About the Breast Cancer Controversy*. New York: Macmillan.

Flexner, M.W. 1947. Cancer—I've had it. *Ladies' Home Journal*, May: 57, 150.

Jones, J. 1993. *Bad Blood: The Tuskegee Syphilis Experiment*. New York: Free Press.

Kasper, A. and S. Ferguson. 2000. Eliminating breast cancer from our future. In *Breast Cancer: Society Shapes an Epidemic*, ed. A. Kasper and S. Ferguson, 355-373. New York: St. Martin's Press.

Klemesrud, J. 1972. New voice in debate on breast surgery. *The New York Times*, December, 12: 56.

Kushner, R. 1975. *Breast Cancer: A Personal and an Investigative Report*. New York: Harcourt Brace Jovanovich.

Lerner, B.H. 2002. Breast cancer activism: Past lessons, future directions. *Nature Reviews Cancer* 2: 225-230.

———— 2001. *The Breast Cancer Wars: Hope, Fear, and the Pursuit of a Cure in Twentieth-Century America*. New York: Oxford University Press.

Lerner, B.H. and B. Rollin. 2001. First, you cry—Twenty-five years later. *Journal of Clinical Oncology* 19: 2967-2969.

Lorde, A. 1980. *The Cancer Journals*. San Francisco: Spinsters.

Oken, D. 1961. What to tell cancer patients: A study of medical attitudes. *Journal of the American Medical Association* 175: 1120-28.

Robertson, N. 1979. A woman's crusade against 'one-step' breast surgery. *The New York Times*, October, 22: section II, 6.

Rollin, B. 2000. *First, You Cry*. New York: Quill.

———— 1980. The best years of my life. *New York Times Magazine*, February: 36-37.

———— 1976a. *First, You Cry*. New York: Lippincott.

———— 1976b. How two women are coping with breast cancer. *Harper's Bazaar*, September: 149, 177, 186.

Rothman, D.J. and S.M. Rothman. 1984. *The Willowbrook Wars*. New York: Harper Collins.

Ruzek, S.B. 1978. *The Women's Health Movement: Feminist Alternatives to Medical Control*. New York: Praeger.

Seaman, B. 1969. *The Doctors' Case Against the Pill*. New York: Peter H. Wyden.

Wilson, J.P. 1974. Mastectomy, yes, but which one? *Journal of the Medical Association of Georgia* 63: 407-409.

CHAPTER THREE

GWYNNE GERTZ

BREAST CANCER:

Dueling Discourses and the Persistence of an Outmoded Paradigm

It is a commonplace in studies of intellectual and professional communities that discourse not only reflects, but also influences practice. One particularly salient instance of this is the influence of the medical profession's discourse on the breast cancer treatment controversy during the middle of the twentieth century. For most of the twentieth century breast cancer discourse and treatment in America has been dominated by the Halsted radical mastectomy. This operation was considered "radical" because of its extensiveness: it not only removed the entire breast but also the pectoralis major and minor (chest) muscles and cleared the axilla (underarm lymph nodes). This en bloc procedure removes muscles that assist arm and shoulder movement and often creates a caved-in chest and a swollen, only partially functioning adjacent arm.

The American surgeon William Stewart Halsted (1852-1922) performed his first radical mastectomy in 1882 at Roosevelt Hospital in New York and it quickly became the standard treatment for breast cancer by 1900. This operation is believed to have the longest life span of any operation performed in America. However, new information came out as early as the 1930s and 1940s about more conservative treatments with equally good results, in conjunction with new information about the systemic nature of the disease that also brought the effectiveness of the Halsted procedure and discourse into doubt. When the operation was finally replaced in 1979 by a more conservative procedure, the modified radical mastectomy, that preserved the underlying chest muscles, there were many questions concerning not only the extraordinary life of this operation, but indeed the lag between new information and new treatment, long after the justification for the operation was called into question. Examining texts from the 1950s through the 1970s, I will focus on the contentious debates and rifts in the medical community at this time between

M.C. Rawlinson and S. Lundeen (eds.), The Voice of Breast Cancer in Medicine and Bioethics, 31-52.

two hostile camps: one that continued to work within an anatomical and mechanistic discourse recognized as "Halstedian" and one that adopted a Bakhtinian dialogized discourse that took into account new scientific information about breast cancer, new uses of adjuvant treatment first advocated in Europe, and perhaps most importantly, the voices and fears of the patients themselves. I will employ Michel Bakhtin's language theories as a lens to better understand the formation of these two discursive communities that appeared to be talking about the same subject during the same time period, but also appeared to operate in two different worlds with two different vocabularies, as I will demonstrate later. In conclusion, I will examine the dangers involved in continuing to uphold "Halstedian" language in current breast cancer discourse and the consequences for women and treatment.

THE HALSTED PROCEDURE: ORIGINS OF A "HEROIC" OPERATION

In the late nineteenth century, doctors believed that breast cancer began as a local tumor of the breast that spread in a centrifugal manner (theory of continuous spread) moving into nearby organs such as the lungs and liver through the lymphatic system without assistance from the bloodstream. Halsted based his radical mastectomy on this belief. He described his elaborate technique in his famous article, "The Treatment of Wounds: Operations for Carcinoma of the Breast" (1891): "About eight years ago I began not only to typically clean out the axilla [armpit] in all cases of cancer of the breast but also, to excise in almost every case the pectoralis major muscle, or at least a general piece of it, and to give the tumor on all sides an exceedingly wide berth" (Halsted 1891, 88). Halsted's radical mastectomy was actually a synthesis of earlier mastectomy operations performed in London, Liverpool, and Philadelphia. Halsted, however, was the first to combine removal of the pectoralis major and minor (chest) muscles with the clearing of the axilla (underarm lymph nodes), along with removal of the breast. Halsted's operation was perceived as a sign of hope in the gloomy area of breast cancer treatment, which at the end of the nineteenth century mostly consisted of palliative measures. At the end of the nineteenth century, breast cancer was considered an incurable disease with tremendous incidence of local recurrence. In 1894 Halsted writes of the grim statistics prior to his operation,

> I sometimes ask physicians who regularly consult with us why they never send us cancers of the breast. They reply, as a rule, that they see many such cases, but supposed that they were incurable. We rarely meet a physician or surgeon who can testify to a single instance of positive cure of the breast. (Halsted 1894, 513)

The rationale for Halsted's belief was that the more he could cut or "clean out," as he described it, the better the chance of getting all the cancer before it had the chance to spread. Halsted says: "But now we can state positively that cancer of the breast is a curable disease if operated upon properly and in time" (ibid.). The Halsted school of meticulous yet radical surgery became vastly disseminated through the country and had a profound effect on the development of modern surgical care in America.

The immense popularity of Halsted's operation in America may be attributed to a variety of cultural, social, and scientific factors that generated a discourse leading to the elevation of surgery as part of a new heroics and new science. There were newly formed venues for self-promotion amongst surgeons such as specialty journals, laboratories, and pathology societies (Morantz-Sanchez 1999). Using the language of the new science helped surgeons establish credentials in the professionalization of medicine. The new study of bacteria in the 1880s, especially Joseph Lister's work on antisepsis, brought forth a confidence that many limitations of surgery could be overcome. With antisepsis and the equally new anesthesia, it was now possible to do more daring and "heroic" surgery. Where American surgeons had formerly been in competition with their preeminent German counterparts, who in fact trained many U.S. physicians, the Halsted was a patriotic "American" procedure. As I will illustrate below, in their discourse, surgeons in the late nineteenth century equated America's political and expansionist power with its surgical power.

During the 1930s new scientific findings began to show that breast cancer spread is not always continuous and that it may be disseminated to outlying lymph nodes by cancer emboli and to other areas through blood channels (Katz 1984, 182). Although these findings starkly refuted Halsted's theory of centrifugal spread, the medical profession largely ignored them and Halsted's operation remained status quo treatment for any woman diagnosed with breast cancer. But in 1952, breakthrough studies by R. S. Handley showed that by the time a breast cancer was detectable for treatment, there was already a 34% chance that growths had already metastasized to the internal mammary nodes, "and where a radical mastectomy was done, it had failed as a curative operation before it started" (Handley 1952, 565). Influenced by such findings, several surgeons, including George Crile, Jr. and Oliver Cope, stopped performing radical mastectomies in the mid 1950s. This period became a time of great contention as evidenced by warring medical discourses concerning breast cancer and treatment. The previously dominant discourse of "attack as quickly as possible and get as much as possible" was based on a description of breast cancer as a local disease that spread in a centrifugal manner. In other words, the very concept of breast cancer was changing: breast cancer was now perceived not as a localized, slow growing disease but as having multiple sites, potentially spreading much more quickly than previously thought, and not only through the lymphatics, but also through the bloodstream—something Halsted believed was not possible. During this period of the breast cancer controversy, Jay Katz describes "voices in the wilderness" creating hostile camps (Katz 1984, 182). Two camps formed, each accusing the other of endangering women's lives. One camp consisted of those who thought that more recent understandings made the Halsted paradigm outdated and opted to try more conservative surgery. This camp, which included surgeons from England, Canada, Scotland, and Scandinavia, employed more conservative procedures and used irradiation as adjunct therapy. The other camp consisted primarily of American surgeons such as Jerome Urban, at

Memorial Hospital, New York, who, in keeping with the Halsted en bloc paradigm, chose to extend the radical operation to a super radical mastectomy.

BAKHTIN'S LANGUAGE THEORIES AND BREAST CANCER DISCOURSE

It is useful to apply a Bakhtinian lens to the languages of these hostile camps in order to understand the roles discourse plays when deeply entrenched relationships of authority are challenged. Bakhtin recognizes a category of discourse of privilege and power that does not need to make sense; it comes, as if from above, with its authority already attached to it. Describing this "authoritative discourse" in *The Dialogic Imagination* he writes,

> The authoritative word demands that we acknowledge it, that we make it our own; it binds us, quite independent of any power it might have to persuade us internally; we encounter it with its authority already fused to it. The authoritative word is located in a distanced zone, organically connected with a past that is felt to be hierarchically higher. It is, so to speak, the word of the fathers. Its authority was already *acknowledged* in the past. It is a *prior* discourse. (Bakhtin 1981, 342; emphasis in the original)

Thus, Bakhtin's "authoritative word" functions to preserve or reproduce discourse. Bakhtin's authoritative discourse perpetuates a "prior discourse" located within a privileged or golden past. And as Bakhtin notes of this "prior," authoritative discourse, it cannot be questioned; it is already in place and must be "recited by heart" (ibid., 341).

But Bakhtin also addresses the ways in which such an official discourse can be played with, thus changing the status of the formerly authoritative word. According to Bakhtin, words do not live singular lives; they brush up against each other, interanimate each other, and acquire new meanings in an *unfinalizable* process. Even if the authoritative word is ultimately agreed with (rather than rejected) it must first, according to Bakhtin, be tested and integrated into one's own framework, so that it becomes partially one's own (Morson and Emerson 1990, 220). In doing so, the authoritative discourse becomes deprived of its absolute authority. Gary Saul Morson and Caryl Emerson describe Bakhtin's "assimilation" as the "process by which the speech of others comes to play a role in our own inner speech" (ibid.). Dialogization occurs because all words *(utterances)* find the object at which they were directed, "already as it were overlain with qualifications, open to dispute, charged with value, already enveloped in an obscuring mist...It [the word] is entangled, shot through with shared thoughts, points of view, alien value judgments and accents" (Bakhtin 1981, 276). As Bakhtin writes about the dialogic nature of language,

> [N]o living word relates to its object in a *singular* way: between the word and its object...is an environment that is often difficult to penetrate. It is precisely in the process of living interaction with this specific environment that the word may be individualized and given stylistic shape. (Ibid.)

In contrast to authoritative discourse, Bakhtin's characterizes an "internally persuasive" discourse that is meaningful for an individual and, unlike authoritative discourse, is a "retelling in one's own words" (ibid., 341-2). It does not come with authority already fused to it; it is persuasive precisely because it makes sense to individuals within their worldview. It is an assimilated discourse.

Bakhtin describes the process by which we play with this already-given language and make it partly our own. By doing so, voices that were not formerly heard can become audible. Bakhtin notes that all words have the "taste" of the contexts in which the word has lived its socially charged life. There is no such thing as a neutral word that belongs to no one. It is "shot through with intentions and actions" of others (Bakhtin 1981, 293). Language

> lies on the border between oneself and the other. The word in language is half someone else's. It becomes "one's own" only when the speaker populates it with his own intention, his own accent, when he appropriates the word, adapting it to his own semantic and expressive intention. (Ibid.)

We live, as it were, on the borders of language. Thus even internally persuasive discourse can and does grow and change for a person, in response to new experiences and by intermingling with other internally persuasive discourses (Bakhtin 1981, 345-6). In other words, formerly internally persuasive discourse can also become less persuasive. It can become distanced—attached to someone else. We may reject older voices and perspectives—in a sense outgrow them. In other words, both authoritative and internally persuasive discourses have the potential for dialogization.

The next section begins by showing how the authoritative discourse of the medical establishment functioned to uphold Halsted and his discourse and to silence the objections of women concerned about losing a breast. But the section then illustrates how the *prior* discourse of the medical establishment becomes, as Bakhtin would state, "entangled, shot through with shared thoughts, points of view, alien judgments" (Bakhtin 1981, 276). Although the most vocal dialogization came into play in the early 1970s, when voices of breast cancer patients interanimated a very public dialogue with members of the medical profession, a more quiet patient resistance appeared prior to the 1970s. It is true that, prior to and during a large part of the 1970s, official medical discourse predominantly admonished women not to consider their vanity before their health, assuming that the two were mutually exclusive. In this authoritative discourse female breast cancer patients who felt that their breasts were valuable components of their identity as women were not taken seriously, as these feelings were deemed frivolous concerns. But in a marvelous example of Bakhtinian reciprocity, particular doctors such as Oliver Cope and George Crile, Jr. began to speak out in women's magazines in the early 1970s. These medical authorities who first spoke out against the Halstedian prior discourse in women's magazines found the life experiences and discourses of their patients to be "internally persuasive."

MEDICAL DISCOURSE: THE AUTHORITATIVE VOICE

The authoritative voice, a prior discourse with its authority already fused to it, can be seen in the language of surgeons who were followers of Halsted. For almost a century the larger-than-life figure of Halsted (both the man and his radical mastectomy procedure) permeated the official or authoritative discourse of breast cancer treatment. Halsted is equated with a late nineteenth-century golden age of surgery and its discourse. In Bakhtinian language it is "prior language" located in a "privileged past" where the heroic surgeon operated with boldness upon the woman's body, which was considered to be a battlefield. This was a period where, as Regina Morantz-Sanchez and others note, new pathological theories and the microscope evolved in interaction with each other, creating the possibilities for new, more extensive surgeries (Morantz-Sanchez 1999, 77). Use of the microscope to diagnose disease became part of the new science. The late nineteenth century thus became an era when the mortality rate from surgery was greatly reduced and both surgeons and patients were more willing to resort to the knife (ibid., 73). This atmosphere paved the way for the popularity of the Halsted radical mastectomy.

Nationalism also played a role in the popularization of the Halsted mastectomy. Christopher Lawrence observes that in the last third of the nineteenth century American surgeons "who had long depended on foreign tutelage and texts, began to extol their national products" (Lawrence 1992, 28). The new radicalness of the Halsted mastectomy also fit perfectly with romantic and grandiose notions of national identity and bold frontier exploration. Thus, the frontier of the West provided explicit metaphors for surgeons to operate on a grand scale. Halsted initially described his radical mastectomy at a surgical meeting in New Orleans in 1898, the year that the U.S., in a move of flagrant nationalism, launched the Spanish-American war. During Halsted's time, surgical metaphors were frequently borrowed from military campaigns. Thus, surgeons became national heroes at the turn of the century.

The Halstedian authoritative discourse could only be questioned with great difficulty—if at all. To do so, as the surgeon George Crile, Jr. later noted, was considered an act of heresy: "When feelings toward a ritualistic procedure like radical mastectomy run so high in a community, it is indeed heresy to consider doing anything less" (Crile 1973a, 67). In 1970 Bernard Fisher commented on this ritualistic discourse when he observed first that radical mastectomy is still, after three–quarters of a century, the most commonly employed surgical procedure in the United States for the treatment of operable breast cancer (Fisher 1970, 4). He then asks,

> How did this come to be? Were [the Halsted mastectomy's] origins so well founded as to justify this unprecedented longevity? Is it really the worth of the operation that has been so vigorously defended against critics over the years or is it, perhaps unknowingly, the eminence of the man who is generally credited with its beginning that is being protected? (Ibid.)

To uphold the Halsted mastectomy was to uphold tradition, with its authority already, as Bakhtin would say, "fused to it." Fisher suggests that this Halstedian tradition and its surrounding discourse were upheld by the medical profession as something given, passed down, and not to be questioned, but not because the reasons for its continuation were necessarily internally persuasive, or "made sense." These were the words of the "father" and the Halsted procedure became part of a sacred discourse.[1]

In the middle of the twentieth century, one camp of surgeons began to vociferously defend the Halsted paradigm and operation in their professional discourse. The importance of upholding the words of the father is forcefully articulated precisely when these words are brought into question. One surgeon, Jerome Urban, created a new, extended radical operation at this time in order to uphold the Halsted paradigm in the wake of new information about the prevalence of early metastasis to the internal mammary nodes. Urban responded to new challenges to the old paradigm of breast cancer spread and treatment with a description of his extended operation, which he described in 1951: "the surgical attack has been extended to include radical chest-wall excision in some highly selected cases" (Urban 1951, 1263). In the same year that R. S. Handley published his new studies of earlier breast cancer spread (1952), Urban performed a new four-to-five hour operation that included the conventional radical mastectomy, but also extended the mastectomy to include the en bloc removal of the chest wall as well as the second, third, fourth, and fifth ribs. During this period, some surgeons went so far as to recommend supraclavicular, or neck, dissection in order to get at more lymph nodes. This operation upholds Halsted's anatomic and mechanistic principles: prominent in Halstedian discourse and treatment is the continued use of an anatomic "local attack" (although extended to more parts of the body) to treat a disease that is beginning to be recognized as systemic rather than local. For Urban successful treatment is less about patient survival and quality of life, and more about the ability to "control." Urban says that, "primary treatment of breast cancer succeeds when the primary tumor and its regional lymph node spread are completely extirpated or destroyed" (Urban 1964, 209). But paradoxically, he also acknowledges that because breast cancer is a systemic disease, "various extensions and refinements of the surgical and radiotherapeutic methods have increased local control significantly, but this improvement has not been as marked in the overall salvage rates" (ibid., 212). In other words, according to Urban, the super-radical operation is successful because it upholds Halsted's principles although it does not necessarily save more lives.

Cushman Haagensen, Director of Surgery at Columbia-Presbyterian Medical Center, also became a prominent voice in the argument to uphold the Halsted paradigm in the wake of new findings by creating a new classification system of patients who he defined as inoperable. Haagensen was greatly influenced by Harvey Cushman at Harvard, who in turn had trained under Halsted at Hopkins (Lerner 2001, 84-5). In other words, Halsted's students became teachers and taught his methods and in doing so handed down his authoritative discourse to the next generation of doctors. In light of new information about earlier internal mammary node spread, Haagensen classified and therefore eliminated approximately half of breast cancer patients as "inoperable," thereby increasing the survival statistics in radical mastectomy. In a bazaar move, Haagensen dismissed the treatment of half the breast cancer patients in order to uphold "the words of the father."

J. Chandler Smith chose to uphold the Halsted paradigm by declaring that survival rates were not valid criteria for determining the success or failure of breast cancer treatment. In his 1956 article, "The Inadequacy of Survival Rates in the Evaluation of Cancer Therapy," Smith's purpose was, like Urban's and Haagensen's, to "reaffirm the principle of [radical] treatment" (Smith 1956, 307). Smith stated that successful treatment could not be determined by survival rates and came to the extraordinary conclusion that dismal survival rates should not interfere with continuing to do the Halsted mastectomy, because a "successful" operation is one that upholds traditional principles (ibid.). Smith ultimately endorsed the view that upholding the Halstedian traditional paradigm, rather than the actual survival of the patient, "should determine the method of therapy" (ibid., 311). Both Haagensen and Smith upheld the Halsted paradigm by redefining the meaning of a term: Haagensen redefined the term "inoperable" and Smith redefined the term "successful" in order to fit the old paradigm. For Smith, Haagensen, and Urban, a successful or superior treatment meant that the largest amount of tumor had been eradicated.

Accompanying these discursive moves was an emerging discourse of breast cancer surgery as a battlefield in which breasts must be sacrificed. If, as Lawrence claimed, surgical democracy "was the frontier of the body, where, surgeons declared, darkness was giving way to light and civilization was taming the 'primary terrors' of pain and suffering" (Lawrence 1992, 30), it is interesting to trace remnants of this type of "heroic" discourse in the writing of surgeons who upheld the Halstedian paradigm and treatment. For example, in 1947 Sir Gordon-Taylor stated, "The spirit of chauvinism still burns within me…I have always allowed my enthusiasm full scope and have more than a dozen times deliberately removed the chain of anterior mediastinal gland along with the internal mammary vessels after resection of the second and third costal cartilages" (Gordon-Taylor 1947, 118). Gordon-Taylor calls this a "truly radical" procedure, thus invoking Halsted's name and legendary status (ibid.). Concerning surgery for Stage 1 and Stage 2 breast cancer (confined to the breast and possibly axilla) he stated, "I have preferred a sharp knife, a stout heart and unquenchable optimism, and have regarded the widest radical surgery untrammeled by ancillary radiation as the method of election in almost every case belonging to these two categories" (ibid.). Gordon-Taylor's language echoes an enthusiastic militarism: the surgeon becomes a soldier who does his conquering with a "sharp knife" and the cancer becomes an insidious enemy that must be taken out, en bloc. What is missing from such discourse is the recognition of an individual and variable body belonging to an actual woman. There is no room in this discourse for new knowledge (which existed at the time) that tumors are biologically variable, and cure of the disease may be more influenced by the aggressiveness of the tumor and the host's (patient's) immune capacities, rather than the surgeon's "derring-do." Such recognition diminishes the activity and primary agency of surgeon-soldier. One can't mix one's metaphors: if the body is a battlefield upon which the surgeon fights the enemy cancer with all his skill and daring-do, then how can the battlefield have her own "will," subsuming that of the soldier's, fighting with its very own immune system the enemy that only the soldier is supposed to be able to engage with? For surgeons such as Smith, Haagensen, Urban, and Gordon-Taylor, who felt the priority of upholding the Halsted paradigm, their militaristic thinking and discourse did not allow for recognition that the host may have any influence on a breast cancer tumor. The individual patient herself seems invisible and without agency.

In this heavily militaristic medical discourse the woman's body is turned over to the surgeon. Her body is a battlefield on which to wage war against the disease. For example, Haagensen advocates the traditional Halsted mastectomy in his book *Diseases of the Breast* (1956) with these words: "Depending upon science rather than art, it [the Halsted mastectomy] is more like a carefully planned military campaign than the painting of a picture" (Haagensen 1956, 587). Although it can be argued that a carefully planned military campaign also takes reason and judgment into consideration, the emphasis is on a pre-planned "rule" for attack. The disease must be fought by the rules of engagement. There is one general procedure for all, rather than individual and variable diseases or bodies. In keeping with this discourse, Haagensen dismisses those who perform more conservative operations as "modern defeatists" who choose to "compromise" rather than give it all they've got (ibid., 657-8).

When surgery is equated with war, the surgeon/soldier is heroic when he is aggressive. Bravery is equated with the amount of potentially dangerous enemy territory removed. To do less is to court defeat in battle. As Haagensen stated in 1960, when cancer has metastasized to the axilla, but is still operable, "the performance of simple mastectomy in a patient who can tolerate a radical operation is nothing less than surgical cowardice" (Haagensen 1960, 82). In the same chapter on radical mastectomy, he writes: "Its performance demands patience and fortitude, and most surgeons are content to do a considerably abbreviated operation" (ibid., 108). Again, less surgery is equated with lack of prowess and fortitude on the part of the surgeon. In a 1967 *Journal of the American Medical Association* article, Haagensen and E. Miller conclude, "Surgery, without question, remains our chief weapon against early breast cancer" (Haagensen and Miller 1967, 150).

In 1960 George Pack and Irving Ariel employed military tropes when they commented on clinical experimentation with radiation and lesser forms of surgery (such as simple mastectomy): "The question arises as to whether there has not actually occurred during this period of therapeutic uncertainty a definite and preventable loss of ground already won" (Pack and Ariel 1960, 4). When Owen Wangensteen and F. John Lewis note the high mortality rate from extended mastectomy they also frame their thoughts within the discourse of war, where one must expect casualties: "However much we would have it otherwise, every war must be fought with the ammunition then available" (Wangensteen and Lewis 1960, 132). And Grantley W. Taylor comments on Wangensteen's super-radical, "I think that the attempts to push forward the frontiers of surgery in all directions are an extremely wholesome thing" (Taylor and Wallace 1950, 843). To do less invasive surgery is a form of defeatism.

When a breast cancer patient's body is defined as a war zone, a woman whose cancer is untreatable has neglected the advance of the enemy and declared defeat. (This may be the one situation where a woman *is* given agency, even though it is in the form of a decisive lack of action, namely, neglect). Thus, in 1943, Frank Adair refers to women who do not fit newly suggested requirements for the Halsted procedure, due to metastases outside of the operable region, as "Primary Inoperable":

> This classification signifies that the patient has neglected her disease until it has passed the breast and corresponding axilla…This represents a neglected case, a case advanced beyond the stage at which the surgeon or the radiation therapist has an opportunity for cure by their respective or combined methods. (Adair 1943, 554)

Due to the woman's negligence, the breast has lost a battle before the surgeon had a chance to attack. This helps to explain why those healthcare workers who thought of breast cancer in terms of military operations (with their call to masculine agency and action) could only perceive new, more conservative procedures in terms of "defeat." Language not only enables and creates possibilities, but also delimits them. Hence a breast, in this militaristic vocabulary, is not recognized as belonging to a woman who may be concerned with aesthetic values. Thus a breast can be removed, but this medical discourse does not allow for any further recognition that the patient may experience physical and/or emotional distress due to the breast's removal.

Perhaps most disturbing in the battlefield metaphor is the way in which a woman's breasts are interpreted as separate from her body. In 1951 George Pack was one of the first to promote bilateral (or prophylactic) mastectomy for all women who have "unilateral" cancer. First, Pack redefined each breast as a combined unit: "In other words, the breasts together should be considered as an anatomic system rather than as separate, unrelated organs" (Pack 1951, 929-30). He based his definition on the fact that both breasts share the same genetic and hormonal factors and possibly etiological factors that influence the development of cancer. Thus, the surgeon redefined breasts as a single unit, one that could then be removed as a package. Pack does recognize there is some conflict of value over the breast's definition: "By a strange paradox, women tolerate the loss of both ovaries [when one is cancerous] better than the removal of both breasts, perhaps because the surgical defects are hidden and not visible as constant reminders" (ibid., 930). But then Pack dismisses these cosmetic concerns,

> The average woman with intact mammary glands believes that two breasts are better than one and one breast is better than none. Except for possible sexual enhancement, there is no valid excuse for retention of the opposite breast if one has become cancerous. It remains largely a nonfunctioning organ and would never be used for nursing a child except under extraordinary conditions. (Ibid.)

Again, in Pack's definition of breasts, they have one exclusive function; otherwise they are "nonfunctioning" and therefore easily dispensable.

Breasts are to be "sacrificed" in war. As Pack writes: "The sacrifice of a useless organ such as the remaining breast therefore does not make the patient a functional cripple as would the complete removal of other paired organs such as the testes" (Pack 1951, 931). Aside from the obvious sexist double standard (viz., refusing to recognize a woman's feelings about her breasts are as valid as a man's feelings about his testes), all value for the breast is equated (by the surgeon) with sexuality. Pack notes with puzzlement that it is extraordinarily difficult to secure consent for bilateral mastectomy when only one breast is involved because even though it would make dressing easier, "[women] cherish the other breast as a token preservation at least of femininity" (ibid.). As a solution, Pack calls for better education of the public and surgeons to help predispose them toward bilateral mastectomy and to help breast cancer patients "overcome this handicap" (ibid.). Note that Pack defines as a "handicap" a woman's valuing of her breasts not only as a part of her sexual identity but as part of her sense of self. Similarly, in the introduction to their 1960 book on the treatment of breast cancer, Pack and Ariel begin by noting the tragedy of women who sacrifice their lives due to an organ "designed for the benefit of the species" (Pack and Ariel 1960, 3). They state, "The situation becomes more tragic in that many women never suckle their young and thereby support an organ which, from a functional standpoint, has deteriorated to being an appendage of questionable ornament from which they may eventually die" (ibid.). In his medical discourse, Pack consistently defines (and limits) what a breast can and cannot signify.

In her book, *A History of the Breast*, Marilyn Yalom notes that men have controlled women's breasts for most of western history (Yalom 1997, 241). Within the medical profession (and its discourse), Yalom describes the "breast" as an exclusively "medicalized breast" where lactation and tumors "have been the major breast-related concerns of the medical profession" (ibid., 239). While Yalom recognizes progress has been made in medical treatment, she also notes, "in the hands of doctors, breasts have been covered with every conceivable concoction, strapped to electric machines, bombarded with radium, squeezed between mammogram plates…and, as a last resort, cut off from the rest of the body" (ibid.). In the authoritative discourse of the medical profession, Pack and others have defined "breasts" for women as either "functional" or "non-functional" and in doing so determine when they may keep them. In accordance with Yalom's critique, surgeons such as Pack continued to assume complete control over the bodies of their patients.

MEDICAL DISCOURSE: THE DIALOGIZED VOICE

Bakhtin's language theories specifically address an "assimilation process" whereby a formerly authoritative discourse becomes *dialogized* and re-accentuated. Bakhtin recognizes the traditional, sacrosanct discourse that "demands we acknowledge it," but he simultaneously recognizes another, alien "internally persuasive" discourse that is "denied all privilege, backed up by no authority at all, and is frequently not even acknowledged in society" (Bakhtin 1981, 342). This second form of "alien" discourse, described by Bakhtin as internally persuasive, precisely encapsulates some of the felt, spoken, but, up until the 1970s, infrequently written about experiences of women with breast cancer. These women's experiences with and concerns about cancer and treatment are subjugated knowledges that have been buried by the authoritative, official discourse. The foreign, (in Bakhtinian terms) "alien," voices of women patients and scientists who described alternate theories to Halsted's theory of tumor spread, "interilluminated," and were incorporated into, the voices of two particular surgeons: Oliver Cope and George Crile, Jr. Both of these surgeons went outside of the medical community and began to write for the popular media in order to reach a wider audience. Crile and Cope chose to appeal directly to women to help put public pressure on a profession they felt to be too insular and resistant to change. As Bakhtin notes, "the semantic structure of an internally persuasive word is not *finite,* it is *open;* in each of the new contexts that dialogize it, this discourse is able to reveal ever newer *ways to mean*" (ibid., 346; emphasis in the original). Cope and Crile took what had been "alien" and assimilated it into their own medical discourse. Oliver Cope, a surgeon at Massachusetts General Hospital, can be seen as an example of a more iconoclastic surgeon, not bound to Halstedian tradition, who interilluminated the voices and fears of patients into his own discourse and in doing so created an alternative discourse about breast cancer and treatment. Cope credits his decision to stop performing Halsted mastectomies in 1960 to both the resistance of patients and more recent medical knowledge. In Bakhtinian terms, he listened to patient's voices that were "denied all privilege, backed up by no authority at all" (Bakhtin 1981, 342) and incorporated these voices into his own discourse and practice as they became "internally persuasive" for him. Cope, like all American surgeons at that time, was trained in the Halsted radical mastectomy from 1928-1932. However, he became dissatisfied and did his last radical in 1960 (Cope 1977) In 1967 Cope and his colleagues presented a paper at a meeting of the New England Surgical Society introducing preliminary data about the selective use of lumpectomy and radiotherapy as alternative treatment at Massachusetts General Hospital. This paper was rejected by the *New England Journal of Medicine* because its contents were deemed too unfamiliar or "alien" for a reputable medical journal. Cope had to go outside of the medical establishment in order to publish the paper: three years later the paper appeared in both the June 1970 issue of the *Radcliffe Quarterly,* the magazine of Radcliffe College, and in a November 1970 issue of *Vogue* (Lerner 2001, 148).

In this article Cope describes several women with breast cancer who came to him prior to 1960 and refused to have the Halsted mastectomy. He then intermingles the voices of patients in his own medical writing. He begins his article with the report of a personally influential incident that took place in 1958. A woman who had a lump in her breast dismissed her surgeon, who planned to remove the breast, just prior to surgery. She requested Cope instead, and he includes parts of her dialogue within his own narrative: "It may seem strange to you, but I have a horror of losing my breast. I am 62, my husband is dead, and I have no thought of marrying again. However, I am still horrified by the thought of losing my breast, and I asked for you [Cope] because I thought you might find a way for me to keep it" (Cope 1971, 264). In the patient's discourse, framed within Cope's narrative, she is not only rejecting traditional treatment but is also, in a Bakhtinian sense, "answering" a prior medical narrative that frequently assumes that women who want to keep their breasts do so exclusively to attract and keep men in an attempt to remain sexually desirable. However, in Cope's narrative, we are presented with a woman who simply does not want to lose part of her body. She is horrified. This is an "alien" voice intercepting the authoritative voice.

Cope recognizes the everyday humanity of his patient's words not only because she expressed her personal fears, but also, as Cope mentions, because he had known her previously as the widow of one of his medical school professors (Cope 1971, 263). Her language became internally persuasive for Cope not only because he was able to hear her voice, but also because he was able to combine it with more recent medical findings. Upon examination, Cope discovered that the woman's breast mass was large, had spread into nearby lymph nodes and "according to the criteria of the day, even radical surgery would probably only delay, and not cure, the disease" (ibid., 264). Cope then recalls that two years prior, another woman in her sixties with a small breast lump had refused to be treated with radical mastectomy. So, Cope had the radiology department treat her with radiation and the patient was "well" and still free of cancer two years later (ibid., 264). Cope refers to new breast cancer research which indicated that the spread of cancer to distant organs may take place much earlier than anticipated and that there is often a wider dissemination of cancer cells in the lymphatic system (particularly to the internal mammary nodes) earlier than previously conceived (ibid., 265). Cope's decision to treat this patient by removing only the lump and using radiation instead of performing a radical mastectomy involved a dialogized thinking process, whereby the words of two patients were interanimated with the words of more recent medical authority within Cope's consciousness. In response to his decision, Cope noted that the general practitioner of his current patient, "was very upset when I did not do the traditional mastectomy, and her son-in-law, also a physician, was outraged at my neglect" (ibid., 264). In the words of these other physicians can be heard the "authoritative voice" that automatically equates "lesser surgery" with defeat in the battle. Even though Cope thought that his treatment methods might be met with disapproval from the more traditional, authoritative members of the medical community, he did not find their reasons for performing radical mastectomies persuasive. As a result, the patient he refers to in this article lived for six more years.

Cope concludes his article by noting the psychological advantage given to women when they have the choice of whether or not to keep their breasts and therefore have a bit more control over decisions involving their bodies. He remarks that it is strange that surgeons have been so slow to realize how women feel about their breasts, and provocatively counters, "only when mutilation is put to [the surgeon] in terms of an analogy—the loss of masculinity—does he react to it" (Cope

1971, 268). Cope's nontraditional medical discourse has been shaped by what Bakhtin would describe as the "internally persuasive" voices of women patients. As Bakhtin writes,

> When someone else's ideological discourse is internally persuasive for us and acknowledged by us, entirely different possibilities open up. Such discourse is of decisive significance in the evolution of an individual consciousness; consciousness awakens to independent ideological life precisely in a world of alien discourses surrounding it, and from which it cannot initially separate itself; the process of distinguishing between one's own and another's thought, is activated rather late in development. (Bakhtin 1981, 345)

The words of patients who refused radical mastectomy were originally "alien discourses" that helped shape new possibilities of treatment for Cope. Unlike Pack, whose discourse defined when a women's breast was worth keeping and when it was merely a "questionable ornament," Cope allows himself to be internally persuaded by the voices and fears of women, including feelings about their breasts. According to Bakhtin, the alien word of another becomes further developed, "applied to new material new conditions; it enters into interanimating relationships with new contexts" (Bakhtin 346). Cope remained aware of the multiple discourses *within* the medical community, along with the internally persuasive discourses of his patients, when he decided to perform his last radical mastectomy in 1960.

Similarly, Cleveland surgeon George Crile, Jr., deemed a heretical figure in the breast cancer controversy from the 1950s through 1970s, employed a discourse that reflected an "interillumination" of alien voices that were, in Bakhtin's terms, "frequently not acknowledged by society" (Bakhtin 342). Crile stopped performing radical mastectomies in 1955 and became an early outspoken critic of the Halsted mastectomy and an advocate for patient's rights who encouraged women to demand information from their doctors about treatment options and become participants in the decision-making process. After 1955, Crile's professional and public discourse reflected his genuine consideration of the fears and preferences of patients in his decision-making.

George Crile frequently expressed concerns in both medical and popular journal articles (Crile 1956, 1961, 1964, 1968) that one of the problems with the Halsted mastectomy was that it actually discouraged women from seeking treatment. These alien voices of refusal were not represented in the authoritative discourse of more established members of the medical community. Crile incorporated into his philosophy and practice and, just as significantly, publicized the findings of a large number of iconoclasts ranging from European surgeons such as Geoffrey Keynes[2] of England and Robert McWhirter of Edinburgh, Scotland, to surgeon/biologist Ian MacDonald, all of whom argued that the Halsted mastectomy was unnecessarily mutilating and should be replaced with a combination of more conservative surgery and radiation. Crile thus helped to shape new theories of how to treat breast cancer effectively.

Crile's writing in the 1950s often began with a dismantling of authoritative Halstedian theories that endorsed the radical mastectomy as the only treatment for breast cancer. In "Cancer of the Breast: The Surgeon's Dilemma" (July 1956), Crile writes that "to date there is no proof that the results of the radical mastectomy are better than those of the simple" (Crile 1956, 179). And since the radical "may cause disfigurement and dysfunction," it must be determined whether this procedure should continue to be routinely employed (ibid.). In this article Crile considers the positive results of McWhirter's[3] work with radiation and simple mastectomy (preserving pectoral muscles and axillary lymph nodes) as an alternative to the radical mastectomy as well as the women who may be "disfigured" and lose functioning in their arm as a result of the Halsted mastectomy. Of McWhirter, Crile writes:

> The chief significance of the [McWhirter's] Edinburgh experiment is that it suggests that in some cases radical mastectomy may *shorten* the period of survival. In all operable stages of the disease, McWhirter found that the results of simple mastectomy were superior to those of radical mastectomy. (Ibid., 180)

Where authoritative medical discourse maintains that radical surgery is the exclusive "weapon" with which to attack the (uniform) disease, Crile speaks of the "disfigurement" and the "disability" that results from the use of such a "weapon." In doing so, Crile changes the battlefield back into a sentient body.

For Crile, not only are breasts part of a body that can be "disfigured" but the cancerous tumor is also an integral part of the body with a "natural course," that must be considered in determining breast cancer treatment options. Early on, he dialogizes his discourse by bringing in the voice of biologist Ian MacDonald, to better understand the behavior of tumors. In an earlier controversial article (1951) on "Biological Predeterminism," MacDonald railed against the prevailing (Halstedian) dogma that the growth rate of all tumors was constant and progressed in an orderly sequence. Instead, MacDonald claimed that the biological nature of cancer is much more complex because there is a great deal of variability in both the growth factor of a tumor and the defensive reactions in the host. In his controversial article MacDonald states that the factors determining the inherent potential of a tumor for growth and dissemination are probably "genetic"; he notes in particular that the failure to improve breast cancer survival rates despite a "drastic increase in the extent of surgical resection" is evidence of "biological predeterminism in cancer of the breast" (MacDonald 1951, 451). When Crile first goes public with an article in *Life* magazine in 1955, he appropriates MacDonald's theory and defines "biologic predeterminism" as "a term that refers to the nature of cancer itself, its speed of growth and its tendency to invade and spread to different parts" (Crile 1955, 132). Thus, Crile defines cancer as a "broad spectrum of disease"; each cancer runs its own course, which is "apt to be independent of tumor size, duration of disease or the type of treatment given" (ibid.). One year later (1956) Crile follows up by publishing an article that applies MacDonald's biologic predeterminism specifically to breast cancer when he writes that the course of breast cancer "is thought to depend chiefly upon the biological properties of the tumor and the resistance of the host" (Crile 1956, 179). The spread therefore depends upon "the resistance of the host and the ability of the circulating cells to implant and to grow [rather] than upon the type of surgical treatment" (ibid., 182). The new theory involved a conceptual transformation in the understanding of breast cancer.

Crile's discourse shifts the focus away from the soldier/surgeon to the individual host (or body), as he observes that it is impossible to prove that any form of surgical treatment influences the course of breast cancer. The individual human being takes priority over standardized generalizations that are applied to all. Crile writes that a patient with breast cancer "should be considered as an individual problem" and that part of the surgeon's challenge is to control the cancer with "the least possible harm" to the patient (Crile 1956, 184). This language emphasizes the individual and the specificity of her body as opposed to articulating a one-size-fits-all-approach to breast cancer treatment.

Crile's goal is to do what is best for the patient. He is concerned with "dangerous operations" that may actually spread disease. Rather than an already-charted military campaign with the surgeon in complete charge, "treatment" is defined as a "delicate balance," where the best treatment is individually based, following decisions made by both doctor and patient together (Crile 1956, 184). There is science here, as Haagensen acknowledges (1956), but this science includes art[4] and not just the weapon of the scalpel.

In his 1955 *Life* article, Crile describes cancer with very different metaphors than Pack's or Urban's:

> Cancer cells are the offspring of our own cells but they are endowed with abnormal properties of growth. Cancer cells *are not invaders from the outside*, not alien creatures that have come to us from some strange form of life. They are, in a sense, our own children gone wrong. (Crile 1955, 132; emphasis added)

The linguistic binary self/non-self does not operate in this discourse. Through non-militaristic metaphors, Crile redefines not only what cancer is, but also emphasizes previously unconsidered options a patient may have when faced with treatment decisions: "Remember that cancer cells are our own cells and they can live side by side with normal cells without causing pain" (ibid., 142). Crile instead discusses quality of life, and the possibility of living with certain incurable cancers that still allow for years of comfort and freedom from pain. He even notes occasions where "inoperable" cancers will mysteriously disappear. Treatment cannot simply be seen as a battle where the surgeon wields a mighty sword. Rather than a military campaign where the body is an area of conquest, good treatment includes a "delicate balance" of the concerns and desires of both doctor and patient.

When Crile wrote for the popular press he was aware of the power of discourse to shape action. In his non-medical writing Crile notes:

> It has been said in the predawn of human history, man became committed to the use of the mechanism of words, with their static meaning, instead of a form which might have allowed him to reproduce more faithfully the fluent character of things as they are. (Crile 1969, 158)

The universe is also joyously messy and unfinalized for Crile. Sounding eerily like Bakhtin himself, Crile continues, "the universe is not static, as our descriptions of it imply, it is not composed of bits and parts, it is dynamic. It flows through space and time" (ibid.). When Crile takes on a word such as *cancer* in his medical discourse, he also asks the reader to consider what qualifies as a "good life," not only in terms of duration but also in terms of personal quality. This discourse is quite different from that which refers to cancer as an enemy or a foreign body that must automatically be eliminated with a "stout heart." Perhaps it is the ability to absorb a multitude of "alien" discourses into one's own voice recognizing, without fear, that meanings are never static or univocal which also permits for that something extra that allows for innovation in the discourse and treatment of breast cancer.

CONTEMPORARY BREAST CANCER DISCOURSE: THE PERSISTENCE OF METAPHOR

Halsted, speaking in 1904 about the unusually tenacious belief in Galen's theory of the four humors,[5] noted: "It is now, as it was then and as it may ever be; conceptions from the past blind us to facts which almost slap us in the face" (Halsted 1904, 371). It is difficult to believe that Halsted would not have been appalled at the longevity of his own operation and the surrounding discourse, after new scientific findings had supposedly dismissed the rationale for such treatment. And yet, today, remnants of this authoritative Halstedian discourse still appear in medical discourse about breast cancer treatment and "blind us to facts" that would allow for the implementation of new knowledge into contemporary discourse and practice.

One contemporary example of resistance to new knowledge can be found in the frequent use of modified radical mastectomies in situations where lumpectomies with radiation have proven just as successful—and in many of these cases, the patients are not informed that there is a treatment choice. For more than a decade, strong evidence has existed that for early stage breast cancer, lumpectomy (removal of the tumor and surrounding tissue only) with radiation is just as effective as the standardized modified radical mastectomy. In 1990 a federal advisory panel stated precisely this, and a more recent October 17, 2002 issue of *The New England Journal of Medicine* confirmed these findings. The twenty-year follow-up of a critical *National Cancer Institute* randomized controlled clinical trial conducted by Bernard Fisher and colleagues, compared early breast cancer patients who had a mastectomy with those who had lumpectomy surgery alone and those who had lumpectomy with irradiation. After twenty years the study showed no difference in survival or recurrence rates between the groups. Among the 1,851 women who participated in the trial, no significant differences were observed with respect to disease-free survival, distant-disease-free survival, or overall survival (Fisher et al. 2002, 1233). And findings showed that lumpectomy and breast irradiation, as compared to lumpectomy alone, actually brought a significant decrease in the incidence of recurrence in the ipsilateral (same) breast (ibid., 1240). This study showed exactly the same thing that former studies showed about the Halsted mastectomy: the extent of local surgical treatment is not the decisive factor in determining the outcome of breast cancer.

Yet the modified radical mastectomy remains the most common treatment despite the findings of these studies (Altman 1992, 190). A doctor writing on breast cancer options in an October 1992 *Vogue* article commented, "Most of those patients who were suitable candidates for lumpectomy [in America] were either unaware of their options or were not offered a choice" (Rosenfeld 1992, 230). By May 19, 1998, Lawrence Altman noted in a *New York Times* article, "Tens of thousands of American women with breast cancer [will be] losing a breast unnecessarily each year" because doctors don't follow national guidelines in treating breast cancer (Altman 1998, 18). The first comprehensive study showed about 65% of breast cancers diagnosed in American women each year are classified as early-stage. Of these, three-quarters are eligible for "breast conserving therapy," which consists of lumpectomy and radiation (ibid.). More than 75% of all tumors can be treated by lumpectomy followed by radiation (Andrews 2003, 12). An editorial by Monica Morrow in a 2002 *New England Journal of Medicine* issue repeats conclusions drawn ten years earlier: "Despite a large body of mature scientific data from randomized trials, which is unequaled in the literature on the local treatment of cancer, many women today are not offered the option of breast conserving therapy" (Morrow 2002, 1270). While it is understandable that a breast cancer patient who is suitable for the operation may prefer not to go through with the intensive adjuvant therapy that comes with lumpectomy—six weeks of radiation for five days each week—it is also clear that, just as in the Halsted mastectomy controversy, many women are simply not given a choice.

Morrow's statement that many women today are not offered the option of breast conserving therapy suggests that too many in the medical profession are still preserving an outmoded, ritualized discourse: "The more you take out the better." As Crile observed about the Halsted mastectomy in 1973, when feelings toward a "ritualistic procedure" [radical mastectomy] run so high in a medical community, it is considered heresy for surgeons to even consider doing anything less (Crile 1973b, 67). The same time lag between knowledge and practice described in detail in the Halsted controversy now appears to be taking place in the lumpectomy controversy, along with employment of similar metaphors and analogies. Doctors and patients still want to "get it all" even though breast cancer is proven to be a systemic, not a local, disease. The "more aggressive" tendencies of American surgeons appear to be firmly embedded in larger cultural beliefs that date back at least to Halsted. In the current lumpectomy controversy, despite decades of "progress," vestiges of Halstedian discourse are still firmly in place. As a result, women continue to pay the physical, financial, and psychological costs of current aggressive, at times outmoded, approaches to breast disease.

It is important to ask larger questions about the possible costs of relying so heavily on an old, authoritative discourse that almost exclusively employs military metaphors to describe breast cancer treatment. An example of this discourse is reflected in one current breast cancer online source that begins: "Before you can launch an effective battle against breast cancer, it's important to understand some basics" (Understanding breast cancer). According to this online source, it seems that we now have laser-guided "smart bombs" that attempt to remove the cancer with less collateral damage: "For well over a century, surgery has been the first line of attack against breast cancer…Today, the goal is precise, targeted surgery that aims to preserve as much of the healthy breast and surrounding areas as possible" (ibid.). But what remains firmly in place is a prominent authoritative medical discourse surrounding breast cancer that tells women to view their cancer exclusively in terms of an enemy from the outside who is colonizing their bodies and must be destroyed.

Our ability to think and discuss events in one way automatically rules out other, competing ways of seeing: you either win a war or you lose, you are either aggressive or you surrender. The metaphors of this militaristic medical discourse not only reflect a way of perceiving breast cancer, but perhaps more significantly, also shape and limit knowledge about both the disease and its "common sense" or "rational" treatment. In other words, the choice of metaphors in medical discourse also determines what will be recognized as valid knowledge. When the focus is almost exclusively on destroying an enemy, other more holistic approaches to preventing and treating disease are interpreted as "alien voices" and are therefore, not taken into consideration. We must begin to ask what sort of information is excluded and what sort of knowledge is deemed "invalid" when militaristic tropes are employed by predominant medical discourse. In what ways might this medical discourse limit healing? How does the focus on destroying the enemy prevent alternative treatment methods from being voiced or heard? How does equating the "enemy" exclusively with cancer blind us to social, cultural, and/or environmental carcinogenic conditions around us that, as Halsted says, "almost slap us in the face"? What is the cost of waging war on a human body? How might "aggressive" treatment procedures be damaging to a patient? And, what role might the human body play in its *own* ability to prevent disease? These kinds of questions have been too often silenced by a militaristic medical discourse that relies on heroic medicine and technology to vanquish the enemy.

Gwynne Gertz received her Ph.D. in English from the University of Illinois at Chicago. She is a Lecturer in the Department of English at the University of Arkansas, Fayetteville.

NOTES

1. Indeed, Mark M. Ravitch began his 1971 talk on the legacy of Halsted's mastectomy before the Johns Hopkins Medical and Surgical Association with these words: "Those who walked these halls before the great burst of surgical and investigative activity which occurred after World War II, started their surgical lives believing that Halsted's collected papers is the 'Good Book' and in it is to be found 'the Word'" (Ravitch 1971, 202).

2. Geoffrey Keynes, of St. Bartholomew's Hospital in London, was one of the first surgeons to advocate less mutilating surgery for breast cancer in the 1920s. He demonstrated that the use of modified radical surgery (sparing the chest muscles) supplemented with radiotherapy instead of the Halsted mastectomy provided equally good survival rates (Keynes 1929).

3. See McWhirter (1948).

4. In a 1964 article on "Early Carcinoma of the Breast," Sir Arthur Porritt also advocates less mutilating breast cancer treatment, noting that the patient with breast cancer "should be treated as a whole, psychologically as well as physically," and concludes his article with a similar rebuttal to Haagensen: "Here, as everywhere else in surgery, there is a human art as well as a progressive science" (Porritt 1964, 216).

5. Clarissimus Galen, the second-century Greek physician, followed Hippocrates' "humoral" theory for disease, which postulated that all illnesses were a result of an imbalance in the four humors, or fluids, in the body: blood, phlegm, yellow bile, and black bile. Galen believed that an excess of black bile caused cancer. His cancer theory became widely disseminated and was not challenged until the eighteenth century. For a more detailed account of Galenic humoral theory, see Olsen (2002).

REFERENCES

Adair, Frank E. 1943. The role of surgery and irradiation in cancer of the breast. *Journal of the American Medical Association* 121: 553-559.

Altman, Lawrence K. 1998. Mastectomy alternative often ignored, study says. *New York Times* 19 May late ed.: A18.

Altman, Roberta and Michael J. Sarg. 1992. *The Cancer Dictionary.* New York: Checkmark Books.

Andrews, Valerie. 2003. Choosing the right treatment. *Mamm: Women, Cancer and Community.* Spring: 10-15.

Bakhtin, M.M. 1981. *The Dialogic Imagination.* Tr. Caryl Emerson and Michael Holquist. Austin: University of Texas Press.

Cope, Oliver. 1977. *The Breast: Its Problems—Benign and Malignant—and How to Deal with Them.* Boston: Houghton Mifflin.

———— 1971. Breast cancer: Has the time come for a less mutilating treatment? *Psychiatry in Medicine* 2: 263-69.

Crile, George Jr. 1973a. Breast cancer: A patient's bill of rights. *Ms.,* September: 66+.

———— *1973b. What Women Should Know About the Breast Cancer Controversy. New York: Macmillan* Publishing.

———— *1969. A Naturalistic View of Man: The Importance of Early Training in Learning, Living, and the Organization of Society. Cleveland: World Publishing Co.*

———— 1968. Results of simple mastectomy without irradiation in the treatment of operative stage 1 cancer of the breast. *Annals of Surgery* 168: 330-336.

———— *1964. Results of simplified treatment of breast cancer. Surgery, Gynecology & Obstetrics* 118: 517-523.

———— 1961. Simplified treatment of cancer of the breast: Early results of a clinical study. *Annals of Surgery* 153: 745-761.

———— *1956. Cancer of the breast: the surgeon's dilemma. Cleveland Clinic Quarterly* 23: 179-184.

———— 1955. A plea against blind fear of cancer. *Life*, October 31: 128+.

Fisher, Bernard. 1970. The surgical dilemma in the primary therapy of invasive breast cancer: A critical appraisal. *Current Problems in Surgery* 3: 3-53.

Fisher, Bernard, Stewart Anderson, and John Bryant et al. 2002. Twenty-year follow-up of a randomized trial comparing total mastectomy, lumpectomy, and lumpectomy plus irradiation for the treatment of invasive breast cancer. *New England Journal of Medicine* 347: 1233-41.

Gordon-Taylor, Gordon. 1947. The treatment of cancer of the breast. *Proceedings of the Royal Society of Medicine* 8: 118-132.

Haagensen, C.D. 1960. Technic of radical mastectomy. In *Treatment of Cancer and Allied Diseases Volume IV: Tumors of the Breast, Chest, and Esophagus,* ed. George T. Pack and Irving M. Ariel, 82-108. New York: Paul B. Hoeber.

———— 1956. *Diseases of the Breast.* Philadelphia: W.B. Saunders.

Haagensen, C.D. and E. Miller. 1967. Is radical mastectomy the optimal procedure for early breast carcinoma? *Journal of the American Medical Association* 199: 739-741.

Halsted, William S. 1904. The training of the surgeon. Bulletin *of the Johns Hopkins Hospital* 15: 267-275.
———— 1894. The results of operations for the cure of cancer of the breast performed at the Johns Hopkins Hospital from June, 1889 to January, 1894. *Annals of Surgery* 20: 497-530.

———— 1891. The treatment of wounds with especial reference to the value of the blood clot in the management of dead spaces. *Johns Hopkins Hospital Reports* 2: 255-314.

Handley, R.S. 1952. Further observations on the internal mammary lymph chain in carcinoma of the breast. *Proceedings of the Royal Society of Medicine* 45: 565-566.

Katz, Jay. 1984. *The Silent World of Doctor and Patient.* London: MacMillan Press.

Keynes, Geoffrey. 1929. The treatment of primary carcinoma of the breast with radium. *Acta Radiologica* 10: 393-401.

Lawrence, Christopher. 1992. *Medical Theory, Surgical Practice: Studies in the History of Surgery.* London: Routledge.

Lerner, Barron H. 2001. *The Breast Cancer Wars: Hope, Fear, and the Pursuit of a Cure in Twentieth-Century America.* New York: Oxford University Press.

MacDonald, Ian. 1951. *Biological predeterminsim in human cancer. Surgery, Gynecology & Obstetrics* 92: 443-452.

McWhirter, Robert. 1948. The treatment of cancer of the breast. *Proceedings of the Royal Society of Medicine* 41: 118-132.

Morrow, Monica. 2002. Rational local therapy for breast cancer. Editorial. *New England Journal of Medicine* 347: 1270-71.

Morantz-Sanchez, Regina. 1999. *Conduct Unbecoming a Woman: Medicine on Trial in Turn-of-the-Century Brooklyn.* New York: Oxford University Press.

Morson, Gary Saul and Caryl Emerson. 1990. *Mikhail Bakhtin: Creation of a Prosaics.* Stanford: Stanford University Press.

Olsen, James S. 2002. *Bathsheba's Breast: Women, Cancer, and History.* Baltimore: Johns Hopkins University Press.

Pack, George T. 1951. Argument for bilateral mastectomy. Editorial. *Surgery* 93: 929-931.

Pack, George T. and Irving M. Ariel. 1960. Treatment of Cancer and Allied Diseases: Volume IV: Tumors of the Breast, Chest, and Esophagus. New York: Paul B. Hoeber.

Porritt, Sir Arthur. 1964. Early carcinoma of the breast. *British Journal of Surgery* 51: 214-216.

Ravitch, Mark M. 1971. Carcinoma of the breast: the place of the Halsted radical mastectomy. *Johns Hopkins Medical Journal* 129: 202-211.

Rosenfeld, Isadore. 1992. Breast cancer: Knowing your options. Vogue, October: 230.

Smith, J. Chandler. 1956. The inadequacy of survival rates in the evaluation of cancer therapy. *Surgery, Gynecology & Obstetrics* 103: 307-312.

Taylor, Grantley W. and Richard H. Wallace. 1950. Carcinoma of the breast: Fifty years experience at the Massachusetts General Hospital. *Annals of Surgery* 132: 833-843.

Understanding breast cancer. 2003. Available at: http://www.breastcancer.org/ubc_intro.html. (Accessed April 2, 2003).

Urban, Jerome A. 1951. Radical excision of the chest wall for mammary cancer. *Cancer* 4: 1263-1285

Wangensteen, Owen H. 1957. Another look at the super-radical operation for breast cancer. *Surgery* 41: 857-860.

Wangensteen, Owen H. and F. John Lewis. 1960. Radical mastectomy with dissection of supraclavicular, mediastinal, and internal mammary lymph nodes. In *Treatment of Cancer and Allied Diseases Vlume IVTumors of the Breast, Chest, and Esophagus*, ed. George T. Pack and Irving M. Ariel, 122-132. New York: Paul B. Hoeber.

Yalom, Marilyn. 1997. *A History of the Breast.* New York: Alfred A. Knopf.

CHAPTER FOUR

LISA DIEDRICH

DOING THINGS WITH IDEAS AND AFFECTS IN THE ILLNESS NARRATIVES OF SUSAN SONTAG AND EVE KOSOFSKY SEDGWICK

In her essay in this volume, Susan Sherwin analyzes the meanings we attach to the experience of illness and suggests that we transform the metaphors available to us to discuss breast cancer. As she notes, "metaphors structure the types of responses we are able to envision as appropriate to a particular domain," and, as such, our choice of metaphors—the ones we choose and the ones available for the choosing—have "ethical significance" (10). Sherwin is concerned in particular with the ways in which the biomedical response to breast cancer is structured by the dominant metaphors used to conceptualize that response. She notes that military metaphors are so dominant that they prevent us from imagining a response that does not require "engaging in deadly warfare, fought on the bodies of women" (12). Sherwin's critique is useful not only in understanding how such metaphors limit the biomedical response, but also in helping us understand how these same metaphors might limit the patient's response to her own illness experience.

If the military metaphors predominate in the biomedical conception of cancer (and I think they do), then a related, and I think similarly limited and limiting response is available to patients: in order to respond "appropriately" to their cancer, they must be "patient" as this battle against cancer is waged on their bodies—that is, according to the *Oxford English Dictionary*'s definition for the adjective "patient,"

> bearing or enduring (pain, affliction, trouble, or evil of any kind) with composure, without discontent or complaint; longsuffering, forbearing; calmly expectant; not hasty or impetuous; quietly awaiting the course or issue of events, etc.; continuing or able to continue a course of action without being daunted by difficulties or hindrances; persistent, constant, diligent, unwearied.

In a sense, then, to be patient is a form of heroism, though it is paradoxically a passive sort of heroism, as opposed to the active heroism that characterizes the

M.C. Rawlinson and S. Lundeen (eds.), The Voice of Breast Cancer in Medicine and Bioethics, 53-68.

doctor's position in the doctor/patient relationship. In fact, one definition of the noun-form of the word "patient" is: "a person or thing that undergoes some action, or to whom or which something is done; that which receives impressions from external agents...as correlative to *agent*, and distinguished from *instrument*; a recipient." *(OED)* What is expected, even required, of persons who are ill is that they perform a passively heroic mode of being ill, while their doctors perform an actively heroic mode of curing.

Like Sherwin, in this essay, I too will not offer "specific advice about the decisions particular women *should* make when confronting the threat or reality of breast cancer in their lives" (5), nor do I mean to suggest that bearing or enduring pain or affliction with composure is a misguided response in the face of a life-threatening disease. Rather, inspired by Sherwin's call to "supplement the dominant framework by developing alternative ways of thinking about health and disease" (16), I want to begin to imagine alternative understandings of breast cancer from the patient's side of the doctor/patient binary. In order to do so, I will consider two illness narratives[1] that attempt to challenge the notion that the most effective way for a person who is ill to respond to his or her illness is to quietly await the course of events as determined by the institution of medicine as it does battle on the patient's body. I will look first at Susan Sontag's discussion of metaphor and illness, and her assertion that all metaphorical thinking must be banished from our response to illness. Although at first glance Sontag's work does not appear to be a personal response to her own experience of illness, I will show that her work might be read as, paradoxically, a depersonalized personal narrative of illness. In fact, Sontag depersonalizes and de-heroicizes her response to illness in order, in her view, to offer a strategy to others that she believes is most *effective* in the face of illness.

Like Sontag, Eve Kosofsky Sedgwick also wants to challenge the passively heroic mode of being ill, but unlike Sontag, she does not believe that depersonalizing that experience is the only or best way to challenge this particular mode of being ill. Making use of her theoretical and political concept of "queer performativity" in relation to her personal experience of breast cancer, Sedgwick not only brings into play a concern for the *effective*, understood as that which is attentive both to the rhetoric and practices of politics, but also for the *affective*, understood as that which is attentive to the poetics and practices of suffering. While both Sontag and Sedgwick offer challenges to the structures and structuring of the experience of illness from the patient's side of the doctor/patient binary, they diverge from each other in their relationship to the affective and its place in their illness narratives. For Sontag, the affective has no place in accounts of illness, and she therefore formulates her challenge to the conventional ways we speak and write of illness in terms of an *intellectual idea that has rhetorical effects*. Sontag believes that by purifying the language we use to speak and write of illness, both of metaphor and of the affective that often gets expressed through metaphor, we will transform the experience of illness itself in necessary ways. Sedgwick, on the other hand, is not interested in purifying the language with which we speak and write of illness, but in queering it, and she formulates her challenge to the conventional ways that we speak and write illness in terms of an *affective experience that has performative effects.* Put succinctly, then, Sontag wants to change the way illness is experienced and narrativized by doing things with ideas, while Sedgwick wants to change the way illness is experienced and narrativized by doing things with affects.

HOW TO DO THINGS WITH IDEAS

In her groundbreaking essay *Illness as Metaphor* (1978), Sontag critiques the social and moral meanings that are attached to certain illnesses; that is, she problematizes the metaphorization of illness and wants to "de-mythologize" disease. To some extent, Sontag's desire to render illness as devoid of moral meanings is not unlike the biomedical approach itself, which attempts to diagnose illness as a pathological fact, an object of analysis for medicine's "speaking eye."[2] Her appeal, however, is patient-centered in that she insists that diagnosis must be of a disease and not of a patient's particular personality or disposition. Sontag attempts, in other words, to purify the experience of illness from normalizing judgments. Tellingly, (though perhaps not surprisingly considering its date of publication) Sontag's work mentions few patients' personal narratives, focusing rather on fictional and medical representations of illness.[3]

By comparing the representations of tuberculosis in the nineteenth century and the representations of cancer in the twentieth century, Sontag suggests that diseases whose etiologies are unknown are most likely to be metaphorized in both medical and popular understandings. In the nineteenth century, according to Sontag, tuberculosis was a disease that was romanticized; that is, it was represented not so much as a debilitating disease, which it clearly was, but as an opportunity for "spiritual refinement" and "expanded consciousness."[4] Unlike tuberculosis, Sontag asserts, cancer has never been romanticized, nor has it been aestheticized. In the twentieth-century representation of cancer, the disease becomes not a reflection of the sufferer's spiritual refinement, but, instead, a reflection of the sufferer's allegedly repressed character. According to such representations, cancer does not expand consciousness, but obliterates it. Sontag, therefore, wants to show that these metaphors—both the good nineteenth-century tuberculosis metaphors and the bad twentieth-century cancer metaphors—are damaging for those persons who are suffering from the actual diseases, which in and of themselves, she insists, do not have moral meanings. Thus, Sontag is impatient with the need to make illness meaningful, even, or especially, by attributing to the experience of illness the impetus to change one's life; that is, to make it meaningful in ways it wasn't before.

Interestingly, considering Sontag's stated de-metaphorizing and de-mythologizing agenda, many commentators on her work have seemingly misread it, and therefore cite only the metaphorical image with which she opens *Illness as Metaphor*:

> Illness is the night-side of life, a more onerous citizenship. Everyone who is born holds dual citizenship, in the kingdom of the well and in the kingdom of the sick. Although

we all prefer to use only the good passport, sooner or later each of us is obliged, at least
for a spell, to identify ourselves as citizens of that other place. (Sontag 1978, 3)

Such emigration/citizenship/national character metaphors have become a recurrent
trope in personal narratives of illness; illness is often referred to as another country
to which one is temporarily or permanently exiled.[5] Which is more useful, then—
Sontag's metaphor or her argument against metaphor? I want to emphasize that
both—the de-metaphorizing idea and metaphorical language—might be useful for
the person who is ill to transform the way illness is experienced and narrativized.

One problem with Sontag's argument is that in asserting that "the healthiest way
of being ill" would be experiencing illness purified of metaphorical thinking, she
retains the health/illness binary characteristic of modern medicine (Sontag 1978, 3).
She seems to be saying, if only implicitly, that there are good and bad ways not only
to be ill, but also (and this is especially important to Sontag) to write about or
represent being ill. In an earlier essay, "Against Interpretation," Sontag asserts that
she wants, and believes it is possible to have, "pure, untranslatable, sensuous
immediacy" in art (Sontag 1966, 9). In the same essay, she explains further that she
is interested in the "sensuous surface of art" rather than in "mucking about in it"
(ibid., 13). We might ask, however, what is the difference between "the sensuous
immediacy" of an experience and "mucking about in it"? I contend that many illness
narratives, in order to describe the sensuous immediacy of illness, must in fact muck
about in it. The "it" that they muck about in is not only the experience of a body
which can no longer be taken for granted, but also the affective responses to that
body as it becomes undisciplined. This is precisely what Eve Sedgwick's work
attempts to do, as I will show in the latter part of this essay.

Sontag's desire for an art that is "unified and clean" is in contradiction, it seems
to me, to her assertion that "[w]hat is important now is to recover our senses. We
must learn to *see* more, to *hear* more, to *feel* more" (Sontag 1966, 14). In the ways
one responds to art as well as in the ways one responds to the experience of illness
(and, of course, the attempt to give this experience of illness form through art),
Sontag is positing the possibility of some prediscursive experience. But,
interestingly, this prediscursive experience, in Sontag's conception, is not unlike
what might be conceived of as an "objective" or "scientific" rendering of
experience: "detached, restful, contemplative, emotionally free, beyond indignation
and approval" (ibid., 27). Sontag is intent on distinguishing the sensual from the
emotional, and asserting that the sensual can be experienced unmediated by either
thought or emotion. Sontag's understanding of aesthetics is related, therefore, to her
understanding of illness and how best to describe it. But, such an understanding, as
Sontag presents it, must leave out the affective voices of patients who use metaphors
to empower themselves to challenge the conventional medical narratives of illness
that emphasize that the patient must be both heroic and passive (or, as I noted at the
outset of this essay, passively heroic) as medicine fights its war on the patient's
body. And yet, via affective misreadings, her work seems to have served as an
inspiration for many people who are ill to write—metaphorically, more often than
not—about their own experiences of illness. Furthermore, Sontag's work has, it

seems to me, most *effectively* de-mythologized disease simply by challenging taken-for-granted representations of illness rather than by successfully purifying the experience of illness of metaphor.[7]

But, as I have presented it thus far, something is missing from my discussion of *Illness as Metaphor*. I have left out a crucial aspect of the book—*the* crucial aspect, perhaps—which is Sontag's motivation for writing *Illness as Metaphor*. Although she doesn't give readers any hint of it in the actual text of *Illness as Metaphor*, there is, paradoxically, a personal story of illness behind her desire to depersonalize the experience of illness. Sontag herself was diagnosed with and treated for breast cancer in the two years before she wrote her treatise on nineteenth and twentieth-century representations of illness. By not mentioning this fact until now, I do not mean to imply that Sontag was in the closet about her cancer, I simply wanted to highlight the fact that her desire to describe the possibility of having a *pure experience of illness* requires that she *depersonalize* her own relationship to illness; it requires that she remove the affective from her explicitly effective analysis.

On January 30, 1978, the same week that the first part of what would become *Illness as Metaphor* was published in *The New York Review of Books*, Sontag was interviewed in *The New York Times*, and the (unnamed) interviewer states, "she makes a point of openness about her illness" (*The New York Times* 1978, A16). Moreover, she herself admits that her own first responses to her diagnosis were not in the form of an idea at all; rather, what she experienced was, "[p]anic. Animal terror. I found myself doing very primitive sorts of things, like sleeping with the light on the first couple of months. I was afraid of the dark. You really do feel as though you're looking into that black hole" (ibid.). In these statements, Sontag attempts to describe the ways in which the person who is ill experiences illness. She attempts, that is, to give her own terrifying experience form in language, and this terrifying experience is given form, at least initially, through metaphor. She *uses* metaphor to explain how illness makes her feel: it is as though she is "looking into that black hole" of her most primitive fears. But, it is important to reiterate that Sontag refuses to reveal this particular affective history both in the text of *Illness as Metaphor* as it was published in *The New York Review of Books* as well as in its slightly revised book form.

Sontag's refusal of the affective leads to some rather ironic readings in at least two of the reviews of the book version of *Illness as Metaphor*. In a review for the *The New York Times*, John Leonard euphemizes Sontag's breast cancer as "[h]er own widely publicized health problems" (Leonard 1978, C19). By speaking euphemistically about cancer, Leonard contributes to the negative ways in which cancer is perceived, which is, of course, precisely what *Illness as Metaphor* argues so effectively against. Despite his vague reference, Leonard nonetheless believes that Sontag's health problems "doubtless account for the tone and content of *Illness as Metaphor*, but they also probably account for its lucidity. It is burned clean of mannerism and of glibness" (ibid.). Leonard's mostly positive review of *Illness as Metaphor* ends with an acknowledgement of both the usefulness of metaphors, in particular as "our way of thinking about death," as well as the necessity for someone, like Sontag, to be a "critic of metaphors" (ibid.). Her credentials to carry out such a task are her experiences both as intellectual—that is, as someone who does things with ideas—and as cancer survivor.

In contrast to Leonard, Denis Donoghue, in *The New York Times Book Review*, doesn't at all like what he takes to be Sontag's angry tone in *Illness as Metaphor*. From his comfortable position outside the kingdom of the ill, he offers a reasoned and reasonable—that is, *not angry*—assertion of his own agency:

> If a doctor gave me a psychological stereotype instead of a cure or an alleviation, I'd demand my money back. If doctors have nothing better to say than that you have cancer because you are the type of person to get cancer, then indeed they should keep quiet. But because they don't know what causes cancer, their offense is venial if they hazard a guess. (Donoghue 1978, 9)

The chasm between doctor and patient in relation to power/knowledge does not worry Donoghue. The passive patient role is not something Donoghue can imagine; he has absolutely no doubt that he would not become passive in that position, but would remain a person and an agent with countless options and the ability to make demands. Despite his own gesture to the personal to dispute Sontag's picture of the doctor/patient relationship, Donoghue suspects that *Illness as Metaphor* "is a deeply personal book pretending for the sake of decency to be a thesis" (ibid., 27). A personal book, Donoghue seems to say, can only pretend "for the sake of decency" to have a thesis. But, as we shall see, Sontag herself will defend against just such a position in her next book about illness. Finally, Donoghue is also not very concerned about the "sinister mythology of cancer" because he cannot believe that it "will persist after the causes of the disease are known and a successful treatment is produced" (ibid., 9). This is precisely Sontag's point, though she recognizes as Donoghue does not, that cancer will not be the last disease with a sinister mythology. And, in just a few years, another disease and its sinister mythology will appear, and Sontag will use this disease as further evidence for her argument.

Ten years after the publication of *Illness as Metaphor*, Sontag returns to her task of de-mythologizing disease; this time her critique is leveled against the rampant metaphorization of the newly discovered and sufficiently mysterious "AIDS virus."[8] What is remarkable about *AIDS and Its Metaphors* (1988) is not so much her delineation of the damaging metaphors attached to HIV/AIDS,[9] but her return to, and, to some extent, rewriting of, *Illness as Metaphor*. For someone "against interpretation," Sontag, surprisingly, offers her own interpretation of her earlier work. We learn, or are reminded, therefore, that Sontag was motivated to write *Illness as Metaphor* not only as a continuation of her work on representation in literature, visual art, and photography, but also because of her own experience with breast cancer. "Twelve years ago," Sontag writes, "when I became a cancer patient, what particularly enraged me—and distracted me from my own terror and despair at my doctor's gloomy prognosis—was seeing how much the very reputation of this illness added to the suffering of those who have it" (Sontag 1988, 12). As I've noted, Sontag's own feelings of terror and despair do not appear in the text of *Illness as Metaphor*. Why not? Because, according to Sontag, as she looks back at that earlier work and time,

> I didn't think it would be useful—and I wanted to be useful—to tell yet one more story in the first person of how someone learned that she or he had cancer, wept, struggled, was comforted, suffered, took courage…though mine was also that story. A narrative, it seemed to me, would be less useful than an idea. (Ibid. 13; ellipses in original)

This is a somewhat strange, though revealing, opposition that Sontag sets up between a narrative and an idea. Presumably, she means specifically a *personal* (or perhaps, affective) narrative because, of course, even her idea must be given narrative form for it to be useful. In *AIDS and Its Metaphors*, Sontag wonders within the text itself what is most useful in the face of illness and, in particular, what is most useful for the person who is ill and others like her.

Sontag, at least at the time she wrote *Illness as Metaphor*, believed that a choice must be made between a personal narrative and an idea. Only later, when writing not about an illness she herself has but about an illness among people she knows and loves, will she feel a need to clarify and put into print the personal motivation that fuelled the writing of *Illness as Metaphor*. And so, in *AIDS and Its Metaphors*, Sontag admits she wrote *Illness as Metaphor* "spurred by evangelical zeal as well as anxiety about how much time I had left to do any living or writing in" (Sontag 1988, 13). But, Sontag explains, "The purpose of my book was to calm the imagination, not to incite it" (ibid., 14), and here, as I will show below, she parts company with Eve Sedgwick, who, as a poet and literary critic, in her work seeks, precisely, to incite the imagination, or, as she might say, to queer it. Although Sontag's demythologizing does question the ways in which illness is represented, her refusal "to incite the imagination" means, it seems to me, that her questioning is somewhat limited in scope. She must rely on ideas that are already available, not thoughts as yet unthought, still to be invented. She must purify the language we use to speak of illness, not invent new languages, as Sedgwick will attempt to do. Sedgwick, unlike Sontag, then, has a literary writer's faith that the inventiveness of language can not only hurt but also help us—that the inventiveness of language, or simply seeking out such inventiveness in language, may in fact be *useful* for those who are living with cancer.

In *AIDS and Its Metaphors*, Sontag wants to prove that *Illness as Metaphor* is a form of what I have called an effective history against the passively heroic position of patienthood; she calls her earlier work "an exhortation" to others to "[g]et the doctors to tell you the truth; be an informed, active patient; find yourself good treatment, because good treatment does exist (amid the widespread ineptitude)" (Sontag 1988, 15). Yet, nowhere in *Illness as Metaphor* does Sontag make such statements, even obliquely. So, why rewrite her earlier work? Why supplement an idea with a personal story of suffering (though brief) and a political exhortation (though belated)? The answer, it seems to me, has something to do with both AIDS and metaphors. That is to say, what Sontag experiences anew in the face of HIV/AIDS is the panic and animal terror that her own diagnosis of breast cancer had brought with it over ten years before. In opening her work on AIDS with a return to her work before AIDS, Sontag seems to doubt the faith she had proclaimed and yet still wants to proclaim: that an idea alone can alleviate suffering, that an idea can illuminate once and for all the black hole of our most primitive fears, that science not emotion is most effective in addressing disease, and that language can and should be purified of the metaphors used to represent those affects—the panic and animal terror—that accompany the experience of illness. With HIV/AIDS the black hole returns, and, although she faces it once more with an idea, there seems to be less certainty that an idea alone is enough.

In contrasting Sontag's illness narrative with Sedgwick's, I wonder if the sequence of illness events has something to do with their differing narrative approaches. In some respects, Sontag's work begins with the personal experience of illness, and yet she is convinced that bringing in this personal experience would undermine the effectiveness of her argument (and Donoghue's review of her work seems to bear this out, though it also shows the ways in which, nonetheless, the personal and affective were read into her work at the time of its publication, just as the metaphorical has been read into it since). Only when her personal experience of illness becomes, paradoxically, also about the personal experiences of illness *of others* does Sontag sense it might be necessary and effective to tell a piece of that personal story, at least as an introduction to her idea now applied to a new illness event. Sedgwick's relationship to the same two illness events experienced by Sontag (breast cancer and AIDS) is reversed. She had experienced the illness of others and written about AIDS before she was diagnosed with and would write about breast cancer. Her political, theoretical, and performative response to AIDS comes before her own experience with breast cancer, but also her ideas about illness emerge out of the affective associated with both AIDS and breast cancer rather than in opposition to it, as Sontag's do.

Before I discuss the ways in which Sedgwick queers the experience of illness and the way we tell that experience, I want to turn briefly to a critique by D.A. Miller of Sontag that reveals the ways in which Sontag's attempt to reduce the affective experience that surrounds illness to an idea diminishes the effectiveness of her argument. Although he is somewhat pleasantly surprised by Sontag's own re-reading of *Illness as Metaphor* and the personal revelations with which she opens *AIDS and Its Metaphors*, D.A. Miller offers a scathing reproach of what he calls Sontag's "urbanity," by which he means her over-intellectualizing, her excessive detachment from any affective response to the crisis of HIV/AIDS, and her focus on exclusively literary as opposed to ethical or political questions. According to Miller, the problem is not Sontag's "'views' on AIDS…so much as in the *attitude of her writing*," that is, "the unexamined and…largely unconscious complex of positionings, protocols, and poses that determine her deployment of language" (Miller 1993, 213; emphasis in the original). Miller's reading of Sontag is important because it points directly to the ways in which Sontag's work itself belies the belated claims she makes for it in *AIDS and Its Metaphors* that I discussed above.[10] Miller recognizes, moreover, that while it may be necessary to oppose certain damaging metaphors—like those associated with the "cancer personality"—it is also possible, and even necessary, to employ metaphor as resistance. Miller, thus, challenges Sontag's concluding "modest proposal" to retire the military imagery attached to illness. Miller finds Sontag's blanket retirement of military metaphors disingenuous at best.[11] According to Miller,

> she forgets how well one such military metaphor—the one conveyed in the word "polemic"...(from the Greek *polemos* [war])—served her as a cancer patient, beset by debilitating myths of "responsibility" and "predisposition." She also overlooks how vital another such metaphor—the one conveyed in the word militancy (from the Latin *miles* [soldier])—is proving to people with AIDS and to the AIDS activism of which they stand at the center. (ibid., 219)

To the terms "polemic" as a form of rhetoric and "militancy" as a form of praxis, we might add the term "queer" as both a form of subjectification and as a form of praxis. As Sedgwick argues, queer is both something we might be and something we might do. In order to understand the ways that we might queer our conception of the passively heroic patient, I turn now to Sedgwick's work, which, although not unconcerned with doing things with ideas, is also concerned with doing things with affects and, in particular, with the affect of shame.

HOW TO DO THINGS WITH SHAME

Along with Judith Butler (1990, 1993a, 1993b, 1997) and Jacques Derrida (1982), Eve Sedgwick has been at the forefront of a move to make use of J.L. Austin's idea of performativity to contest essentialist notions of identity in general and of gender and sexuality in particular. In their introduction to the collection *Performativity and Performance* (1995), Sedgwick and Andrew Parker begin with two questions that emerge out of their reading of J.L. Austin's *How to Do Things with Words* (1961)[12]: "When is saying something doing something? And how is saying something doing something?" (Parker and Sedgwick 1995, 1). A performative utterance, according to Austin, is that which enacts something in the moment it is spoken. One example of a performative that Austin gives, and Butler, Parker and Sedgwick, and others have elaborated on quite extensively, is the statement "I do [take this man or woman to be my lawfully wedded husband or wife]." In saying "I do" one becomes something one wasn't in the moment before the saying: husband or wife (presuming, of course, that the social context for this performance is, in Austin's terminology, "felicitous"). What many commentators on Austin have noted, and which Austin himself makes much of, is that many things can go wrong in the performance of a performative making that performative "infelicitous" or "unhappy"; in other words, as Austin also asserts, a performative can become "ill" (Parker and Sedgwick 1995, 3; Austin 1961, 18-19). In their reading of Austin, Parker and Sedgwick place the possibility—or, indeed, the inevitability—of a performative becoming ill at the center of the notion of the performative: they note, "illness [is]...understood here as intrinsic to and thus constitutive of the structure of performatives" (Parker and Sedgwick 1995, 3). Thus, according to Parker and Sedgwick, "a performative utterance is one, as it were, that always may get sick" (ibid.). In their discussion, Parker and Sedgwick then move from the possibility of an "ill" performative to the somewhat analogous notions of a "perverse" or "queer" performative in order to discuss the notion of performativity in relation to the example of "the Pentagon's 1993 'don't ask, don't tell, don't pursue' policy on lesbians and gay men in the U.S. military" (ibid., 5). I want to move the other way—back from "queer" to "ill"—in order to make use of Sedgwick's concept of "queer performativity" for understanding and narrating the experience of patienthood.

I will begin by delineating what Sedgwick means by "queer" before determining the ways in which a queer performative might be useful in relation to the experience of patienthood, and putting that experience into "language and action."[13] In her collection of essays entitled *Tendencies* (1993b), Sedgwick explains that "something about *queer* is inextinguishable," and defines "queer" as:

> A continuing moment, movement, motive—recurrent, eddying, *troublant*. The word "queer" itself means *across*—it comes from the Indo-European root *–twerkw*, which also yields the German *quer* (transverse), Latin *torque* (to twist), English *athwart*....The immemorial current that *queer* represents is antiseparatist as it is antiassimilationist. Keenly, it is relational, and strange. (Sedgwick 1993b, xii)

Queer, for Sedgwick then, is a continuing movement across bodies and differences. It is at once relational—it perceives beings in relation—and strange—it doesn't attempt to make anyone's gender or sexuality "signify monolithically" (ibid., 8).

In her essay "Queer Performativity" (1993a), Sedgwick discusses the plethora of recent uses of Judith Butler's notion of performativity, and worries that such uses are "a sadly premature domestication of a conceptual tool whose powers we really have barely yet to explore," because they all generally reach the same conclusion: that a particular performance is "really *parodic and subversive* (e.g. of gender essentialism) or just *upholds[]the same status quo* " (Sedgwick 1993a, 15; emphasis in the original). Sedgwick wants to go beyond these dichotomous good performative/bad performative formulations, and in an attempt to use the concept of performativity (from both Butler and Austin) more radically, she explores it as a means of

> understanding the obliquities among *meaning, being,* and *doing*; not only around the examples of drag performance and (its derivative?) gendered self-presentation, but equally for such complex speech acts as coming out, for work around AIDS and other grave identity-implicating illnesses, and for the self-labeled, transversely but urgently representational placarded body of *demonstration*. (Ibid., 2; emphasis in the original)

At this point in Sedgwick's work, the experience of illness, not the rhetorical notion of an ill performative, becomes a means by which one might imagine a more radical form of performativity, or indeed, a specifically queer form of performativity. Although for Sedgwick the concept of queer emerged specifically out of her work on gender and sexuality, she recognizes how useful—personally, politically, and theoretically—it might be, where AIDS as well as her own breast cancer are concerned, to have those experiences of illness confront the theoretical models that had helped her "make sense of the world so far":

> The phenomenology of life-threatening illness; the performativity of a life threatened, relatively early on, by illness; the recent crystallization of a politics explicitly oriented

around grave illness; exploring these connections *has* (at least for me it has) to mean hurling my energies outward to inhabit the very farthest of the loose ends where representation, identity, gender, sexuality, and the body can't be made to line up neatly together. (Sedgwick 1993b, 13)

For Sedgwick, exploring the connections (and disconnections) between modes of being ill, the meanings attached to illness, and the politics surrounding illness (that is, between forms of meaning, being, and doing that surround the experience of illness), requires that she hurl her energies outward into new forms of representation and embodiment, rather than, as Sontag proposes, inward into a "pure, untranslatable, sensuous immediacy" (Sontag 1966, 9). Sedgwick doesn't expect this confrontation to create a work that is "unified and clean," as Sontag aspires to. Rather, it is only in "mucking about in" the panic, terror, and other affects attached to the experience of illness that one might invent new forms of being patient, and new languages for representing that experience.

For Sedgwick, one affect in particular—shame—will connect the two illness events—AIDS and breast cancer—that (although not always the explicit focus of her work, nonetheless) haunt much of it.[14] In many respects, Sontag too is responding in her work to the shame that accompanies patienthood, but she responds by attempting to do away with this shame by arguing that illness has nothing to do with who a person is. Sedgwick believes, on the contrary, that illness does in fact have something to do with who one is, and she responds by attempting to do something else with the shame that is experienced along with illness. For her, shame is an affect that produces and delineates identity, usually a stigmatized identity: "Shame, as opposed to guilt, is a bad feeling that does not attach to what one does, but to what one is" (Sedgwick 1993a, 12). Shame is used to manage identity, and, moreover, though Sedgwick does not mention this specifically, it is used to manage desire as well. At the same time, however, shame can be a "near-exhaustible source of transformational energy," an "experimental, creative, performative force" (ibid., 4). Shame is, in fact, not only productive of normalizing identifications, but it is also productive of transgressive disidentifications. Sedgwick wants to make the shame that one experiences along with illness creative of new ways of being and doing.

In her own illness narrative "White Glasses," the final essay in *Tendencies*, Sedgwick writes about both AIDS and breast cancer; in fact, she recognizes that there is a "dialectical epistemology between the two diseases" (Sedgwick 1993b, 15). This "dialectical epistemology" has emerged out of the history of the two illness events in the West. As Sedgwick notes, the AIDS activism that emerged in the 1980s was influenced by the women's health movement of the 1970s, which encouraged women to become experts on their own bodies and to challenge their objectification within the institution of medicine with new knowledge and new de-institutionalized practices of health care. In turn, according to Sedgwick, "an activist politics of breast cancer, spearheaded by lesbians, seems in the last year or two to have been emerging based on the model of AIDS activism" (ibid., 15). This dialectical epistemology between AIDS and breast cancer is not only demonstrated through the activism surrounding these diseases, but also in terms of "the kinds of secret each has constituted" and "the kinds of *out*ness each has required and inspired" (ibid.). Sedgwick wonders how shame has operated on those who are ill with AIDS and breast cancer, and how that shame has been a source of new forms of outness. For Sedgwick, the two diseases have "made an intimate motive for me," a phrase that I believe reveals in its odd locution Sedgwick's definition of "queer" as movement across, as relational, and as strange. How can we create intimacy out of illness—across bodies and across differences—and how can that intimacy be a motive to create new forms of embodiment and representation?

"White Glasses" opens with a confession of sorts about how Sedgwick in setting out to write the piece "got everything wrong" (Sedgwick 1993b, 255). As she discovers, she got everything wrong simply because she thought the difference between health and illness and between living and dying was clearly demarcated, that those categories were, as Sontag might say, "unified and clean":

> When I decided to write "White Glasses" four months ago, I thought my friend Michael Lynch was dying and I thought I was healthy. Unreflecting, I formed my identity as the prospective writer of this piece around the obituary presumption that my own frame for speaking, the margin of my survival and exemption, was the clearest thing in the world. In fact it was totally opaque: Michael didn't die; I wasn't healthy: within the space of a couple of weeks, we were dealing with a breathtaking revival of Michael's energy, alertness, appetite—also with my unexpected diagnosis with breast cancer already metastasized to several lymph nodes. (Ibid.)

It is impossible, Sedgwick discovers, to make this narrative unified and clean; instead, she must get everything wrong, and yet still attempt to move across the binaries between health and illness, living and dying, between Michael's identity (as a gay man) and her own identity (as a straight woman). This position of getting everything wrong doesn't paralyze Sedgwick with shame; rather, it allows her to create identifications across difference, and, even, "across the ontological crack between the living and the dead" (ibid., 257). According to Sedgwick, it is "exciting that Michael is alive and full of beans today, sick as he is; I think it is exciting to both of us that I am; and in many ways it is full of stimulation and interest, even, to be ill and writing" (ibid., 256). It is exciting to both Lynch and Sedgwick that she is what exactly? Sick? Alive and full of beans today? Sick *and yet* alive and full of beans today? Or, simply, that she is? Here Sedgwick leaves open rather than closes down (or purifies) the affective that permeates her own experience of illness, which is always also more than hers alone. Moreover, a crucial aspect of this is leaving open the possibilities that might emerge out of the relationship between being ill and writing.

Although Sontag's work is effective in challenging the normalizing judgments attached to the experience of illness, it is less effective in challenging the binary relationship between health and illness. She successfully critiques the troubling metaphors used to describe the experience of illness, but does not consider questions of how to live as a person who is ill.[15] Sedgwick is concerned with precisely this, and she recognizes that she is fortunate to be surrounded by models for how to live as a person who is ill. This is, in fact, one thing she has learned and continues to learn from Michael Lynch:

So much about how to be sick—how to occupy most truthfully and powerfully, and at the same time constantly to question and deconstruct, the sick role, the identity of the "person living with life-threatening disease"—had long been embodied in him, and performed by him, in ways which many of us, sick and well, have had reason to appreciate keenly. (Sedgwick 1993b, 261)

Two of the many lessons that Sedgwick learns from Michael Lynch are also two examples of a queer performative: "Out, out" and "Include, include." These queer performatives induce persons living with life-threatening illnesses,

to entrust as many people as one possibly can with one's actual body and its needs, one's stories about its fate, one's dreams and one's sources of information or hypothesis about disease, cure, consolation, denial, and the state or institutional violence that are also invested in one's illness. (Ibid.)

Sedgwick believes that "transformative political work" can be done by making oneself "available to be identified with in the very grain of one's illness (which is to say, the grain of one's own intellectual, emotional, bodily self as refracted through illness and as resistant to it)" (ibid.). Yes, ideas are useful in the face of life-threatening disease, but so are stories, dreams, and hypotheses about the panic, terror, shame, and the institutional violence that we endure and resist. To queer the experience of patienthood is to "include, include" not to "purify, purify."

Lisa Diedrich is Assistant Professor of Women's Studies at Stony Brook University.

NOTES

1. I take the term "illness narratives" from psychiatrist Arthur Kleinman's important work, *The Illness Narratives: Suffering, Healing, and the Human Condition* (1988). Kleinman's book describes the ways in which illness takes on personal and cultural meanings, as well as the ways in which illness and its meanings are given narrative form. He focuses, in particular, on the ways that narrative helps to bring order and give coherence to the experience of illness (Kleinman 1988, 49). I use the term here to refer to published accounts of the experience of illness, though Kleinman, in fact, does not look at published accounts of illness experiences. Rather, he employs an ethnographic methodology and offers ethnographic case studies that demonstrate the multiple meanings that surround illness, especially chronic illness.

2. I take the concept of the "speaking eye" from Foucault's "archaeology of medical perception," in *The Birth of the Clinic* (1973). In that work, Foucault diagnoses the emergence of what he calls the "anatomo-clinical method" at the end of the eighteenth century. According to this method as Foucault describes it, language and the gaze converge on an object: the pathological fact extricated from the patient's body. The ideal of convergence between language and gaze is that of a "speaking eye" that provides an "exhaustive description" (Foucault 1973, 113). "Description in clinical medicine," Foucault explains, "does not mean placing the hidden or the invisible within reach of those who have no direct access to them; what it means is to give speech to that which everyone sees without seeing—a speech that can be understood only by those initiated into true speech" (ibid., 115). In this domain, therefore, the patient is not capable of true speech, even though she may speak of her illness; rather, she is the ground upon which this initiation—the doctor's initiation—takes place. Like the disease itself, the patient's words are objects to be interpreted by the doctor, to be translated by the doctor's "speaking eye" into a pathological fact, and incorporated into a case history.

3. In her groundbreaking work *Reconstructing Illness* (1993), Anne Hunsaker Hawkins uses the term "pathography" for illness narratives, and she defines pathography as "our modern detective story," where we are transported out of the everyday, familiar world of health into the unknown, uncharted world of illness (Hawkins 1993, 1). Hawkins asserts that, as a genre, pathography "seems to have emerged ex nihilo; book-length personal accounts of illness are uncommon before 1950 and rarely found before 1900" (ibid., 3). I contend that the emergence of the women's health movement's challenge to the institution of medicine in the 1970s, as well as feminism's more general assertion that the "personal is political," are contributing factors to the recent popularity of this genre. The emergence of HIV/AIDS in the 1980s, the influence of the women's health movement on AIDS activism, and the fact that HIV initially affected so many people involved in the arts (at least in the gay communities hit hardest in the United States) also seems to have contributed to the rise of this particular genre.

4. I should note that Sontag doesn't really comment on the transformation of the representations of tuberculosis in the twentieth century. Once the tubercle bacillus was discovered in 1882, and once it became known in 1943 that it could be treated successfully with antibiotics, tuberculosis became a less mysterious disease. It also became de-aestheticized, as it became associated with the poor and immigrant populations living in the tenement squalor of large cities. The fact that Sontag doesn't address twentieth-century representations of tuberculosis, however, doesn't contradict her general argument about moral meanings attached to illness; rather, it confirms that such moral meanings are not ahistorical.

5. For example, in his recent book on what he calls "postmodern illness," David Morris uses the first two sentences of Sontag's image as the epigraph for his chapter entitled "The Country of the Ill" (Morris 1998, 21). In his book, Morris discusses Sontag's work at length and is not at all confused about her argument, but, nonetheless, he finds her metaphoric image as compelling as her anti-metaphoric idea.

6. Thanks to Cindy Patton for this insight.

7. And, in this regard, Sherwin's work, and mine too, might be read as a continuation not an overturning of Sontag's critique.

8. The mystery of this particular disease is partly revealed in the complicated history of its naming. The term "AIDS virus," though technically inaccurate, came into common parlance in the early years of the disease. Once the HIV virus was identified, the phrase "HIV, the virus that causes AIDS," was seen more frequently. In her recent book, *Globaliżng AIDS* , Cindy Patton notes in a footnote that "[m]any clinicians and researchers consider HIV to be a 'spectrum' disease; that is, there are a range of manifestations of different degrees of severity" (Patton 2002, 134). She also notes that where HIV/AIDS is concerned there is a "shifting sand of definition...further complicated by the pressure from disability and health insurers, who wanted clear guidelines for who should be covered under their programs. Activists entered the fray in contradictory ways, seeking more rapid research on drug treatments, which might be aided by strict clinical definitions, but also seeking to expand the definitions of AIDS to include more, rather than fewer, affected people in social programs" (ibid., 135).

9. Some, like D.A. Miller (1993), as I will discuss below, claim Sontag actually contributes to rather than critiques these damaging metaphors.

10. It is important to note that Miller is most troubled by the fact that Sontag wants to "move beyond the specifically gay bearings of AIDS metaphors" (Miller 1993, 214). Therefore, he argues, contra Sontag's attempts to de-homosexualize AIDS, that AIDS is "the disease of gayness itself," which is precisely the sort of metaphorization that Sontag would find so troubling. What does Miller seek in pressing so desperately for AIDS to remain centrally a gay disease? By emphasizing the gayness of AIDS, he believes that he might also emphasize its potential political and personal effects. But,

ironically, this itself is a rather urbane politics that circumscribes the potential affinities that might emerge out of the reality of AIDS, affinities beyond AIDS and its gayness. Sedgwick, as I will show below, reveals some of the possibilities that arise out of the formation of affinities between persons with AIDS and persons with breast cancer. Nonetheless, Miller rightly, it seems to me, decries Sontag's attempts—as a writer—to remain "unsituated" and "impeccably detached" (ibid., 216).

11. This is a critique that Sherwin is aware of in her essay in this volume. She acknowledges that the military metaphors might be useful for some, but also insists that by relying solely on such metaphors, we are limiting the inventiveness, and thus potentially the effectiveness, of our responses to illness.

12. *How to Do Things with Words* is a posthumous publication of a series of lectures that Austin gave at Harvard in the 1950s.

13. In her important work on breast cancer that was published just after *Illness as Metaphor*, Audre Lorde calls for the "transformation of the silence" surrounding the experience of breast cancer into "language and action" (Lorde 1980, 20).

14. For example, her most recent work, *A Dialogue on Love* (1999), is a memoir about the relationship between doctor and patient in psychoanalysis. Sedgwick begins analysis after experiencing depression as a result of her diagnosis of and treatment for breast cancer. Sedgwick has also written an afterword to Gary Fisher's illness narrative, *Gary in Your Pocket* (1996), in which she considers critically her role in editing and publishing Fisher's work after his death from AIDS.

15. This relates, I think, to Foucault's late work on ethics in which he contrasted the notion of a fixed gay identity with the more open possibility of trying to define and develop a gay way of life. In an interview for the French magazine *Gai Pied* that appeared in April 1981, Foucault describes how this might work: "Homosexuality is a historic occasion to reopen affective and relational virtualities, not so much through the intrinsic qualities of the homosexual but because the 'slantwise' position of the latter, as it were, the diagonal lines he can lay out in the social fabric allow these virtualities to come to light" (Foucault 1997, 138).

REFERENCES

Austin, J.L. 1961. *How to Do Things With Words*. Cambridge, Massachusetts: Harvard University Press.

Butler, Judith. 1997. *Excitable Speech: A Politics of the Performative*. New York and London: Routledge.

——— 1993a. *Bodies that Matter: On the Discursive Limits of Sex."* New York and London: Routledge.

——— 1993b. Imitation and gender insubordination. In *The Lesbian and Gay Studies Reader*, ed. Henry Abelove, Michele Aina Barale, and David M. Halperin, 307-320. New York and London: Routledge.

——— 1990. *Gender Trouble: Feminism and the Subversion of Identity*. New York and London: Routledge.

Derrida, Jacques. 1982. *Margins of Philosophy*. Tr. Alan Bass. Chicago: University of Chicago Press.

Donoghue, Denis. 1978. Disease should be itself. *The New York Times Book Review*, July, 16: 9, 27.

Fisher, Gary. 1996. *Gary in Your Pocket: Stories and Notebooks of Gary Fisher*. Ed. Eve Kosofsky Sedgwick. Durham and London: Duke University Press.

Foucault, Michel. 1997. Friendship as a way of life. In *Ethics: Subjectivity and Truth,* ed. Paul Rabinow, tr. Robert Hurley, 135-140. New York: The New Press.

———— 1973. *The Birth of the Clinic: An Archeology of Medical Perception.* Tr. A.M. Sheridan Smith. New York: Vintage.

Hawkins, Anne Hunsaker. 1993. *Reconstructing Illness: Studies in Pathography.* West Lafayette, Indiana: Purdue University Press.

Kleinman, Arthur. 1988. *The Illness Narratives: Suffering, Healing, and the Human Condition.* New York: Basic Books.

Leonard, John. 1978. Books of the times: *Illness as Metaphor. The New York Times*, June, 1: C19.

Lorde, Audre. 1980. *The Cancer Journals.* San Francisco: Aunt Lute Books.

Miller, D.A. 1993. Sontag's urbanity. In *The Lesbian and Gay Studies Reader*, ed. Henry Abelove, Michele Aina Barale, and David M. Halperin, 212-220. New York and London: Routledge.

Morris, David. 1998. *Illness and Culture in the Postmodern Age.* Berkeley: University of California Press.

The New York Times. 1978. Susan Sontag found crisis of cancer added a fierce intensity to life. January, 30: A16.

Parker, Andrew and Eve Kosofsky Sedgwick, eds. 1995. Introduction. In *Performativity and Performance*, 1-18. New York: Routledge.

Patton, Cindy. 2002. *Globalizing AIDS* . Minneapolis: University of Minnesota Press.

Sedgwick, Eve Kosofsky. 1999. *A Dialogue on Love.* Boston: Beacon Press.

———— 1993a. Queer performativity: Henry James's *The Art of the Novel. Gay and Lesbian Quarterly* 1, no.1: 1-16.

———— 1993b. *Tendencies.* Durham: Duke University Press.

Sontag, Susan. 1988. *AIDS and Its Metaphors.* London: Penguin.

———— 1978. *Illness as Metaphor.* New York: Farrar, Straus and Giroux.

———— 1966. *Against Interpretation and Other Essays.* New York: Anchor Books.

II. NARRATIVES OF BREAST CANCER:
LIVING WITH DISEASE

CHAPTER FIVE

ANITA HO

THE BREAST CANCER DIARIES

June 10, 2003

I haven't read my horoscope for a long time now. When I was a teenager, reading the horoscope was the entertainment of the week. I would look into the newspaper and find the horoscope for Cancer. I remember reading that Cancer is symbolized by the Crab, and that the body parts that are associated with this sign are the breasts. How ironic it is that I am right now worrying about breast cancer.

I have heard that women should have monthly breast examinations. But at the age of 31, that seems unnecessary. Besides, I don't smoke, drink, or even eat meat. And didn't I read somewhere that Asians have lower chances of getting cancer?

Today I thought it was time to have a self-examination. I suppose it is like flossing before going to the dentist. I have a physical examination with my doctor next week, and if she asks if I conduct monthly self-examinations, I can "honestly" say that I just started doing that.

But this little lump in my breast makes me wish that I had started the monthly self-examination earlier. Maybe I'm not doing it right. I followed the illustration on the self-examination card, but I wonder if still photos really help that much. Perhaps we all have lumps. But why have I never noticed this lump before? Does this mean I have breast cancer? Am I dying? I can't die now! I am not even tenured yet! Besides, I can't die before my parents and grandparents! It is considered a curse in the Chinese culture for children to die before their parents.

Okay, maybe I am paranoid. I look up various Internet sites for more information. Many articles note that most women have lumps in their breasts, and that eighty percent of these lumps are non-cancerous. Some of them also mention that Ashkenazi Jews and people with a family history of cancer are at higher risks. Well, I am not Jewish. I also don't recall any relatives talking about having cancer, although now I wonder what those mysterious surgeries that my great aunts and my dad's sister had were all about. Even though my training in bioethics reminds me

71

M.C. Rawlinson and S. Lundeen (eds.), *The Voice of Breast Cancer in Medicine and Bioethics*, 71-88.

that the traditional medical assumption of genetic differences among ethnic groups is flawed, I find myself holding on to the idea that Asians have a lower rate of cancer occurrence than other ethnic groups. Moreover, statistics show that women at the age of 30 only have 1 out of 2500 chances of having breast cancer. Although I am usually a pessimist, I doubt I will be *that* unlucky this time.

I tell Carl,[1] my partner, about the lump. "Do you think this feels weird?" I ask. Carl sees me touching my breast, and immediately assumes that it is an invitation to sex. "I would be more than happy to give you a breast exam," he says, with a big smile on his face. He tries to fondle me, and I keep asking him to just focus on the lump. He finds the lump, and acknowledges that it feels a bit strange. However, instead of being alarmed, he keeps kissing and stroking me. I try to tell him that I am worrying about my mortality, but somehow Carl does not seem to catch on.

June 26, 2003

I went to my doctor last week, and she gave me a clinical breast examination. She told me that I should not worry. She assured me that given my age and lack of confirmed family history, my lump is probably benign. But just to be certain, she recommended that I have a mammogram and ultrasound.

Although I have taught students about various ethical issues surrounding the process of genetic testing for BRCA1 and BRCA2 in my bioethics classes, I have not paid much attention to the mechanics of mammography. Most of my friends are in their late 20's or early 30's, so we don't usually sit around and talk about mammograms. I asked my mom about it, but she didn't want to discuss anything about breasts. So I asked my sister-in-law, who is a nurse, and she said, "Just imagine slamming the refrigerator door on your breasts."

My mom and Carl came with me to one of the local breast centers. Mom flew here from Hong Kong a couple days ago for a visit, although her vacation plan is unrelated to my "lump discovery." At first I thought Mom should just stay home and rest, since I don't expect the mammogram to take too long. However, she thought it would be easier to come with me, since she wants to go shopping with me afterwards. She wants to buy some presents for her friends in New York—we are visiting them there next week.

The nurses and therapists here seem quite nice. It is as if they're trying to be as nurturing as possible before slamming the refrigerator door on me. My radiation therapist, Michelle, takes me to a brightly lit room with a big machine. She keeps calling me "dear" and "honey," perhaps to comfort me, and maybe to indirectly ask me not to get upset with her when she slams the "fridge door" on me later. "You will feel a bit of discomfort, honey," she says, "but I promise this won't take long. Just hold your breath while I take the x-rays."

Standing stiff in front of the mammogram machine with one of my arms up, I can hear the "fridge doors" coming toward me. Unfortunately, I can't simply open the "fridge doors" and release myself. I am clamped tight and there is no way to get out.

After repeating the process a few times on both of my breasts, Michelle tells me that I can have a seat and relax. "I will take these films to the radiologist and be back in a few minutes."

Sitting alone in the brightly lit room, I stare at the cold and sterile mammogram machine. I realize that this block of steel has probably saved many women's lives, but the tight clamping was certainly no healing touch.

A few minutes later, Michelle comes back in. "We need to take a few more slides because we couldn't see clearly enough from the previous films," she says. I start to feel suspicious—I wonder what exactly they are trying to see. And I wonder if I have to pay for all those "unclear" slides.

When Michelle finally finishes the mammogram, she leads me to the ultrasound room across the hallway. The ultrasound room is cold and dark, but the whole process seems easy enough. Being able to lie on the padded examination table after the torturous mammogram is a bonus—it allows me to relax and recover from the trauma. The warm gel on the transducer gently rolling on my skin is almost soothing, a big contrast to the cold and heavy plates slamming on my breasts. And it is nice to look at the ultrasound monitor. I don't really know what the technician is looking for—I only see that she keeps putting little marks of "x" on edges of various gray areas. However, having the monitor right there gives me the feeling that I am in control, since I get to see what is happening in my breasts.

"So, what exactly are you looking for?" I ask the technician, who never told me her name. "We are trying to see if your lump is a cyst or a tumor," she responds stoically while she wraps up the examination. "The radiologist will tell you more about it."

As I wait impatiently to put my clothes back on so I can keep myself warm, a radiologist comes in with a folder in his arm. "Hi, I'm Dr. Farrell. So, I heard that you came in because you found a lump," Dr. Farrell says. "Well, it looks like the lump is benign. It is just a cyst." Good. Maybe I can put my clothes back on and not freeze in here!

"Oh, but don't change yet. I want to show you these slides. Something perked our interest." *Interest!* What does that mean? It sounds like a euphemism that helps the doctor break the bad news.

Dr. Farrell takes some slides out of the folder and puts them on the light box. "Can you see these little specks on the mammogram? This is a cluster of calcification."

"What does that mean?" I ask. "Didn't you say that the lump is benign?"

"Yes. Forget about the lump. It's fine. I'm talking about something else. We found some clusters of calcification in this other place. At this point, they are undetectable to the human touch and cannot be seen by the naked eye. You won't even be able to feel them. However, the jagged edges of these specks are often an indication of early-stage cancer."

Still sitting on the padded table with the gown on, I stare at the films and wonder what this all means. Dr. Farrell asks if I have any questions. "I don't know what to ask. I thought I came in to confirm that I *don't* have breast cancer!"

"Well, we don't know for sure yet, but on a scale of 1 to 5, 5 being most likely to be cancerous, I would say that this cluster is between 4 and 5. Dr. Davran will meet with you in a few minutes. He will be your surgeon, and he can give you more information about surgery options and other treatment possibilities. Michelle told me that your family came with you this morning. Maybe they can join you in Dr. Davran's office."

I did not even know that I had an appointment with a surgeon. And they already checked out who came with me to the clinic. Do they think I need emotional support? This can't be good.

Still in the hospital gown, I walk to Dr. Davran's office. He confidently introduces himself to me. His bright smile makes me feel cautiously optimistic. "Do you want your family in here, so they can also hear about this?"

I sense that Dr. Farrell has already spoken to Dr. Davran. Although I still don't know what exactly Dr. Davran is going to tell us, I agree to let both Mom and Carl come in. I haven't seen them for almost an hour, and they both look concerned. They perhaps also realize that if they are called in, things are probably not good. Mom closes her eyes and mumbles to herself—I think she might be saying some sort of prayer.

The small examination room is getting crowded, and it feels suffocating. Dr. Davran explains that I probably have DCIS, or ductal carcinoma in situ. I have never heard of this, so he draws a diagram to illustrate what that means, and where the cancer may be. "This is actually good news, at least in the sense that this is an early stage breast cancer. We suspect that the cancer has not spread. This is serendipitous! If you hadn't found a lump, you would not have come in, and we would not have discovered this other site that might be cancerous. So you are very lucky!"

I don't know if one can say I'm lucky or that this is serendipitous. Being the 1 out of 2500 doesn't sound lucky to me—I am now a statistic. But Dr. Davran's sincerity and tone of optimism make me want to believe him.

"Well, open your gown, and let me show you where we found the calcification." I embarrassingly open my gown, fully aware that Mom is also in the room. Mom also feels awkward of looking at my breasts in front of two men—she glances for a couple seconds and then lowers her head to stare at the floor.

When Dr. Davran puts his finger on the right side of my right breast to point out the cancer site, I express my confusion. "This just sounds very strange, especially since I did not feel a lump there."

Continuing on his theme of luck, Dr. Davran says, "That is why you are very lucky. If you did not have the other lump, your general practitioner probably would not have ordered a mammogram because of your age. We would not have found out about the possible cancer. If left unnoticed and untreated, this could develop into a big lump in a couple years, and that might be too late. This is really the best-case scenario, if you can actually say that in this type of situation.

"So, here is what we are going to do. We will try to do a core needle biopsy. We'll take some samples from the site and see if there is any cancer. If so, we will decide what to do."

I ask Dr. Davran how the biopsy works and if it will hurt. He smiles and says, "I haven't heard anyone screaming, so it can't be that bad. Besides, it will only take a few minutes." I appreciate his humor and feel relieved, especially after the painful mammogram.

If only Dr. Davran had breasts and could have tried this himself before telling me that the biopsy does not hurt! The therapist I met earlier, Michelle, is once again attending to me, and she looks even more apologetic than before. "Oh honey, I am sorry that you have to do this. I'll make this quick, okay?" She asks me to lie down on this strange-looking table with a hole. "Place your right breast through the hole, dear. I will pull your breast down through the hole, so that the radiologist can position it with the compression paddle. But don't worry. The paddle has less pressure than the mammogram."

The problem for me isn't so much the compression paddle, but the pulling and yanking of the breast in the attempt to place the breast in the right position. "Ouch! Do you really have to pull this hard?" "I'm sorry, honey. The machine is designed for women with larger breasts, and since you are smaller, this is a bit difficult. Just hold on for another minute, okay?" I don't understand why engineers haven't designed a machine that can accommodate women of all sizes. Michelle's constant sighing also starts to make me feel guilty. While I am sure that she is not blaming me, I begin to feel that I am making her job more difficult by having smaller breasts.

If the mammogram is like slamming a fridge door on the breast, the process of getting the biopsy ready is like pulling a stuck doorknob. I am in so much pain that I have no energy to speak up or to even try and convince Michelle to stop. Maybe that's why Dr. Davran believes that the biopsy cannot be that bad, since no one screamed. I think the clinic simply has a good soundproofing system; or maybe they are all in denial.

After a few minutes of torture, Michelle finally gives up. "I am really sorry for having you go through all that for nothing, but I just have to stop, or I might pull your breast off! You might want to get dressed and meet with Dr. Davran to talk about a surgical biopsy. Sorry, dear. I hope that you won't get too many bruises from this."

"So, that didn't work, hey?" Dr. Davran tries to be lighthearted about it, but I'm still in too much pain to laugh about it. I want to tell him that I did not give any "informed" consent to the process—I did not really know what to expect before I lay down on the table. I also want to tell him that if he really wanted to understand the whole process, he should have the technicians simulate the procedure on his penis. But since he might be the one operating on me, I better just keep my mouth shut.

"Well, we will need to have a surgery to take out some samples to see if there is cancer as we think there is. Hopefully we can get all the cancer out in the first surgery. But if not, we may have to perform further surgeries. And after your surgery wounds heal, you will receive radiation treatment. Most studies on DCIS are done on women much older than you are, so we don't know for sure that radiation will work in your case. But it is worth a try, since it has minimal risks. If the cancer ever comes back, I would recommend a mastectomy. But let's not worry about that right now. I will refer you to an oncologist and a radiation oncologist, and they can explain all that to you at a later time."

Multiple surgeries and radiation that may not even work? Possible mastectomy in the future? Why do I suddenly have so many doctors? It is easy for him to say that I should not worry about that right now. As of a couple hours ago, I thought I was only coming in to confirm that I do *not* have cancer.

Dr. Davran continues. "With the lumpectomies and radiation, the breast with cancer will shrink a bit. So be prepared that the two breasts may look a bit lopsided and asymmetrical."

What? Lopsided breasts? As a feminist, I have always tried to fight various oppressive norms of what women's breasts should look like. But, I have never planned on showing my breasts to strangers. Suddenly, the whole idea of having scars and lopsided breasts started to bother me.

Dr. Davran is probably thinking that I am foolish and vain, and that I should worry more about my mortality than my appearance. "Many women have asymmetrical breasts anyways," he says.

Just when I want to tell him that I don't remember seeing any celebrities with lopsided breasts, Dr. Davran gives me a wake up call. "So, let's book a surgery date. How about tomorrow? Are you free? We can get this done right away."

Tomorrow? Either I have the best insurance plan or they think I am dying.

I know that my health care coverage isn't all that great.

June 27, 2003

Sitting in the pre-op area, I am exhausted and worrying about my first surgery. I did not sleep well last night. More than 45 million Americans have no insurance whatsoever. Many people are on long waiting lists for essential medical services, and some of them die before they receive any treatment. If the hospital is taking me in right away, they must think I am in trouble. I keep trying to think about the big picture as I attempt to process all of the information about my situation. However, since I only learned about the surgery and possible cancer less than twenty-four hours ago, I am still lost in terms of what this all means.

Mom also seems nervous, and Carl tries to comfort both of us. Mom keeps mumbling about how she thinks I got cancer. "If you had listened to me, this wouldn't have happened. I have told you many times that microwave food is dangerous," she says while shaking her head. "And you really should eat meat again. Being a vegetarian is just unhealthy." I want to tell her that I need her to stay calm and not blame me, but it seems that she needs to let it out. "You aren't supposed to have breast cancer at your age. It may be the bras that you have been wearing—I don't think they give enough support." I wonder how Mom knows what kind of bras I have been wearing, but I am afraid to ask. Mom has always been body conscious, but I don't feel like fighting over bras right before my breast surgery. I try to explain that there might be some genetic factors that relate to breast cancer, and ask her about her aunts who had some major surgeries about ten or fifteen years ago, but Mom does not want to talk about them.

Finally, a nurse calls my name and takes me to a small waiting booth. An anesthesiologist greets me and explains the use of anesthesia, and then asks me to sign an informed consent form to certify that I understand the risk of death. Gosh. Why even bother to have the surgery if I might die either way! More importantly, why didn't they tell me yesterday about the risks with anesthesia? What is the point of telling me these risks right before the surgery?

I reluctantly sign the form, and secretly pray that this will not be my last signature. Since we are married, I also wonder if Carl would still have to pay all my medical expenses if they botched the surgery.

Finally, Dr. Davran comes in to tell us that he is ready to take me into the surgery room. On my way to the surgery room, I have a flashback of the movie *Dead Man Walking*. I have never had surgery before, and this all seems surreal. It is as if I were walking to the death chamber, except that I don't have a nun by my side praying for me. Dr. Davran notices that I look a bit pale and asks how I am feeling. "Well, I have been better—I just signed an informed consent form to certify that I know I might die! I know I might be paranoid, but could you make sure that I don't become a case study? I don't want any of my students to read about my case in their textbook!" At the back of my mind, I keep thinking about a case at a local hospital, where a woman went through a double mastectomy a few months ago only to find out that she never had cancer. The lab that did the test mixed up her chart with another patient's.

"Don't worry. We will take care of you."

The six magic words. *We will take care of you.* With these comforting words, I drift away.

July 1, 2003

Dr. Davran kept his magic words. I did not die.

Right now I am in New York City. I probably should have stayed home, but Mom and I have planned this vacation for months. We have never gone on a trip alone before, especially since we now live on different continents. This was supposed to be a chance for us to get together, relax, and visit with her friends. She hasn't seen these friends for ten years, and it seems to be a shame to cancel the trip. Besides, when you are on Vicodin, you think you can do anything.

Mom is superstitious and does not want anyone else to know about my situation. She thinks that if other people know about it, I will be surrounded by bad energy and it will make things worse. She also does not want to talk about anything relating to breasts, especially damaged breasts. In fact, even dad doesn't know about this yet. Mom says she will tell him when she returns home.

Mom wants to get a few gifts for her friends and Macy's in Manhattan seems to be the perfect place. After all, it is the biggest department store in the world.

While Mom is looking at some gift packs, the phone rings, and it startles both of us. Mom drops the merchandise, and waits for me to answer the phone. The caller-ID shows that it is a call from the clinic where Dr. Davran works. I suspect he is calling to tell me about the lab results. However, I don't really want to take the call in front of Mom, in case it is bad news. "I'll be right back, Mom. Just keep looking."

Fortunately, it is easy to find a small corner in the world's largest department store and be hidden from everyone else. I walk into a corner in the lingerie department—Mom would probably feel too embarrassed to come into this section.

"Hello," I say, and wait for Dr. Davran to say, "*Good news!*"

Instead, he says, "Hey! This is Dr. Davran! How is New York? When are you coming back?"

I am pleased that he remembers about my trip. That shows that he pays attention to his patients and truly listens to them. Nonetheless, his question alarms me. "When *should* I come back?"

"Well, the results came back, and you have DCIS, which is what we thought and talked about." He makes it sound like I should have expected it.

"The cancer is of high grade, but the good thing is that it hasn't spread. We found cancer cells very close to the margins of the specimen, which means that we might not have got all of the cancer. We need to do another operation and hopefully we will get it all this time. Can I book you in for tomorrow?"

I can feel my heart pounding, and my tears start to flow uncontrollably. Maybe I should have expected it, but I was still hoping for the best. Another operation tomorrow? How bad is this?

"I am coming back tomorrow night. Can we wait?"

"Sure. I will book you in for the day after," he says. "The important thing to remember is that the cancer has not spread. So this is good news."

I don't know how this can be good news when I need to have another surgery right away. While I know that he is trying to be optimistic, I start to resent that Dr. Davran keeps saying that "this is good news," or that I am "lucky." Is he just saying these things so that I will not scream at him or break down while talking to him? I know that Dr. Davran is trying to be reassuring, but every time when I hear that I am lucky, I feel that I am being selfish and arrogant to be sad about my own situation.

Then I see Mom looking around for me by the bras. She must have followed me after I left. She does not seem embarrassed by the lingerie collections around her; she seems concerned. She is trying to get some clues from my facial expression.

I tell Dr. Davran that I will book the surgery time with his nurse. Even though I have lots of questions for him, such as what it means when he said the cancer was "high grade," I quickly get off the phone and wipe off my tears. I walk over to Mom, and joke a bit about getting a better bra with push-up pads for the smaller breast. She does not seem amused, and asks if I just spoke to Dr. Davran. I tell her the "good news," that the cancer has not metastasized. Then I add that since the margins aren't clear, they want to perform another surgery to make sure that they get everything.

Mom seems suspicious with my response, and she looks very concerned. She keeps saying that it does not sound good, as if I needed a reminder. I want to cry, scream, simply curl up on the floor, be comforted, and have someone else feel sorry for me, but I find myself trying to comfort Mom instead. "This is actually the best-case scenario, Mom, since the cancer hasn't spread. Dr. Davran said that I am very lucky to have found out about this so early."

While I may not have convinced myself that I am lucky, Mom starts to calm down a bit. She then realizes that we are still in the lingerie department and wants to leave. "Why don't you go to the food court while I call Carl? My cellphone probably won't work in the basement level, so I will call up here, and then meet you downstairs." Anxious to leave the bra area, Mom is happy to comply.

I try to compose myself and call Carl. He comes on the phone after the first ring. As soon as I hear his voice, I break down again. "Oh no!" he says. Even though I haven't said a word about what Dr. Davran told me, Carl can tell I don't have good news. While he is worried, as an optimist, he tries to sound calm. "Don't worry, sweetie. I have been doing a lot of research on the Internet. You can read all the information when you come back tomorrow, but I think we will be okay. I feel so bad that I'm not there with you!"

Even though he tries to comfort me, I cannot help but realize that he is more than a thousand miles away, and I feel alone and small in the world's largest department store.

July 23, 2003

I survived my second surgery. Dr. Davran told me that this time the margins are clear—they did not find any cancer cells around the margins. He once again reminded me that I was lucky. However, he suggested that I should have radiation treatment to lower my chance of recurrence and to kill any remaining cancer cells that might still be in my breast.

I have my first meeting with the oncologist, Dr. Coleman, to discuss my treatment options. The waiting room area is full of patients, most of whom are elderly people. Some of them look sickly, and a couple of them sit in wheelchairs and have hats on. I am probably the youngest patient in there.

Dr. Coleman's nurse calls my name. She brings me to a consultation room and asks me to change into the hospital gown. I look around the small room with simple clinic furniture. On a small bare desk, there is a little business card holder. I expected to see Dr. Coleman's cards in there. Instead, the cards read: "*Julie Stevens—Patient Advocate.*"

Just when I am puzzling over why we need other patient advocates besides doctors and nurses, Dr. Coleman walks in. He is probably not much older than I am, but he looks tired. He is quiet, reserved, and looks too serious for a young oncologist. I don't know if he is the best technician in the world, but judging from his demeanor, he does not care about me or my situation.

Dr. Coleman sits down, and places my unopened file on his desk. "So, tell me what brings you here." I wonder why I need to answer this question for yet another doctor. Don't they read the files? I thought Dr. Davran had already talked to Dr.

Coleman about my condition, and that he had sent him my pathologist's reports. It is ironic that in the age of healthcare teams, my care is fragmented. Each professional member is only responsible for one aspect of my care, and no one knows what the others are doing. I simply tell Dr. Coleman that I found a lump and had two surgeries, and that the margins are clear from the second surgery.

Dr. Coleman nods and stares at the floor silently. Just when I am about to ask him when I should start my radiation treatment, and whether I should take hormonal treatment at my age, he looks up with a blank face and says, "Well, even though they think that your margins are clear, you should take that with a grain of salt. Actually, take it with a block of salt. I'm not trying to doubt the pathologists, but to be brutally honest, they don't investigate every single cell when they look at the specimen. So there really is no guarantee that there is no cancer left."

He is right; he *is* brutal. *Take it with a block of salt?*Has he read my file? If he is trying to make sure that I don't feel too hopeful about my prognosis, he certainly is succeeding. I can feel my eyes swelling up. "Well, I just want to know if I am going to be all right. I'm not going to die, am I?"

"The radiation hopefully will cut down your chances of recurrence, and kill any remaining cancer cells that the pathologists may not have found. Hormonal therapy such as Tamoxifen post radiation may help some older women, but I don't know if they would help you at this point. DCIS is very treatable, but I just want to make sure you know what it means when they said that the margins were clear."

I wonder if that's what Dr. Coleman thinks of his professional requirement of truth-telling. Certainly, doctors should be honest with their patients, but could he not have conveyed the truth more gently? I have looked up many medical sites, and Dr. Davran had given me information, also. I knew that surgeries would still not guarantee that there wouldn't be any cancer cells left. I recognized that given my occurrence of cancer at such an early age, I have a substantial chance of recurrence. I also knew that most of the studies on breast cancer treatments were done on women much older than me, and so the results regarding treatment benefits may not apply to me. Even though Dr. Davran was always positive (perhaps too positive), he never told me that there was any guarantee. But somehow when Dr. Coleman asks me to take anything hopeful with a block of salt, I feel as if he is hitting me with a block.

Dr. Coleman gives me the name of my radiation oncologist (Dr. Feber), and tells me that she will give me more information regarding radiation therapy. I glance at my file, which remained closed throughout the whole consultation. On his way out, Dr. Coleman asks me to speak to the receptionist to make a follow-up appointment.

After he closes the door, I start to sob, and wonder how I can continue to see this doctor. He may be the best clinician in the world, but he seems to have no communication skills. Certainly, the requirement of informed consent demands that doctors be truthful with their patients. However, instead of giving me concrete information and helping me make choices based on my overall values, the *brutally honest* oncologist has not given me much information. Instead of feeling empowered to make an informed decision regarding my treatment by his truth-telling, I feel isolated and overwhelmed.

I only hope that Dr. Feber has better communication skills with her patients. As many bioethicists have noted, how physicians communicate and present information has a significant impact on patient care. It is ironic that when technologies are helping more and more patients live longer, physicians' poor communication skills can make patients feel less hopeful.

Wiping off my tears, I once again notice the business cards on the small desk. I pick one up and put it in my pocket—we need patient advocates after all!

August 7, 2003

I met Dr. Feber last week to get some information on radiation therapy. She recommended that I start the therapy as soon as my surgery wounds heal. I am still confused about whether I truly need or should have radiation treatment. Most studies on the benefits of radiation treatment for breast cancers are done on post-menopausal women. Moreover, my sister-in-law, who is a nurse in Vancouver, told me that doctors in Canada usually do not prescribe radiation treatment after surgery for DCIS. I wonder if the different treatment recommendations are the result of varying payment systems in the two countries or different professional opinions on the medical benefits of radiation. I cannot help but wonder if my doctors would have recommended the same treatment if I didn't have insurance.

When I mentioned the different treatment patterns to Dr. Feber, she did not offer any theory. She simply said that in her professional opinion, I could benefit from radiation therapy. So today I am back to the clinic for my treatment-planning session.

"You are just too young to be here!" Sandie, one of my radiation therapists, says sympathetically. "I bet you were shocked when you first found out about your cancer."

I keep wondering if I should sound upbeat in my conversations with Sandie. It has been a while since I first found out about my condition, so I have had some time to understand and get used to the whole situation. Nonetheless, I can't say I want to be here—I still feel a bit overwhelmed about the radiation treatment that will take place every weekday for the next eight weeks.

I am also worried about my medical costs. When I moved to the United States from Canada less than three years ago, I signed up for the cheapest insurance plan my college had to offer. At the time, I was relatively healthy, and having been taken care of by the Canadian universal health care system, I was reluctant to pay a high monthly premium for my insurance. I therefore chose the cheaper plan with the higher deductible and maximum out-of-pocket payment. Although no one has said anything about the costs of my treatment, the fact that every facility asked me for my insurance card before they inquired about my drug allergies reminds me that I will bear some substantial financial responsibility for my treatments.

Feeling awkward telling Sandie about my anxiety, I simply let her do the talking and try to look as upbeat as possible. "You seem to be taking all this quite well," Sandie says. "Your emotional strength can be important in helping you through the whole process." I smile, and decide not to point out the irony.

After the small talk, Sandie takes me into the simulation room. "The treatment machines we will be using for the next seven weeks will be identical to the one here, so you will get a sense of what the treatment will be like."

Sandie gives me a hospital gown. "Just change into the gown and make yourself comfortable," she says. "Dr. Feber will look at your mammograms, and then we will take some x-rays to plan your treatment."

It is difficult to feel comfortable in this cold room with a big machine, and once I get out of my clothes and into the gown, I just sit on the simulation table. I can see Sandie talking to Dr. Feber and a couple other therapists in the next room. They are looking at some films and pointing at various places in those films. I assume that those are my mammograms and they are discussing my treatments. I don't know why they can't discuss them with me there. After all, these are *my* films, and they're planning *my* treatment.

Sandie turns around and sees that I am already sitting on the simulation table. She signals Dr. Feber and the other therapists, and they come into the simulation room to greet me.

"We were just looking at the mammograms," Sandie says. "We want to take some x-rays and measure your tumor site. Just lie down on the table and we will help direct your body to fit the machine. Be very still, okay?"

Lying on the simulation table with the gown open in the front, I feel a chill going through my body. I can hear and see the machine moving over my head. Sandie and Dr. Feber look at my breast and measure the location of my tumor, while the other two therapists observe and take notes. "It looks like your scar is starting to heal quite nicely," Dr. Feber says. I wonder if this is supposed to be another piece of good news and whether I should thank her for her "compliment."

It feels awkward having four strangers surrounding me, probing and staring at my breast. It's as if I'm on a stage experiencing the glare of the spotlight. They all focus intensely on my breast and scar area, and keep talking to each other in codes and medical jargon. Perhaps they don't think that I need to know what they are saying, since *they* are the ones with the medical training who are planning my treatment. However, I thought that medical care in 2003 is supposed to be patient-centered. Hearing them talking to each other as if I were not there makes me feel like a mannequin with movable body parts.

A ruler is placed on my scarred breast numerous times, and the therapists take turn to measure my surgery site from various angles and record a few numbers. "Ninety-six-point-five," Sandie says at one point. I have no idea what that means, but since I am supposed to be as still as possible, I guess I shouldn't talk to them, in case I move.

I can see beams of light coming from the ceiling and out of various machines. Although I am lying down, I can see my own reflection in the tilted windows on the observation booth at the end of the room. Those beams of light all point at my breast, particularly around the scar area. It is a bit surreal; by virtue of my reflection I watch helplessly as laser beams seem to attack my body, leaving it fragmented and broken. "Don't move, okay? We need to mark your skin, and that will help us position you each time you come in for your treatment." Guided by the laser beams, Sandie carefully draws a cross on my upper chest, and then places a transparent tape over it. She then draws another line below it, and places another tape over the second mark.

I continue to lie still, wondering if the cross can keep me safe. Still staring at my reflections in the tilted windows, I can see that I am marked and labeled.

September 8, 2003

"So, how are things? Do you have any questions today?"

Dr. Feber asks the same questions every week during my check up. Every Monday, they take a couple x-rays right before my treatment, and Dr. Feber meets with me right after my treatment. I don't know why they take x-rays every week, but since they have not told me anything, I assume that they have not found anything suspicious from the films. Dr. Feber is a minimalist when it comes to communicating with me. She is gentle, reserved, and aloof. I want to have more of a conversation with her every week when I meet with her, but she does not have much to say. She is not rude or insensitive, as in the case of Dr. Coleman. She just does not concern herself with how I feel. She also doesn't seem to think that she needs to tell me anything unless I ask her, but the problem is that, most of the time, I don't have any questions. Or, I should say, I don't know what to ask. Last week I didn't have any questions, and Dr. Feber simply said quietly, "I won't keep you then. Have a good week, and I'll see you next Monday."

I have tried to discuss various treatment prospects with Dr. Feber. However, since her specialization is in radiation treatment, she does not feel comfortable answering questions not directly related to radiation therapy. When I asked her about Tamoxifen, a hormonal drug that shows promise in many post-menopausal breast-cancer patients, she simply told me to get more information from Dr. Coleman. I wanted to tell her that I would rather not go back to him, but I didn't know if it would be professionally appropriate for me to complain about one doctor to another.

I received some type of healthcare statement a few days ago, and now I wish that I had asked more questions during my weekly checkups. I am still not used to maneuvering through all of these medical statements in order to figure out which portion of the cost is my insurance company's responsibility and which part of the cost I'm going to have to pay. Sometimes I receive letters that say, "This is not a bill." Other times I get statements with astronomical figures but no clear indication of whether I have to pay the full amount. In any case, why do they still charge $483 for every "consultation" when sometimes I don't have any questions and they don't tell me anything? And why do I always have to come up with my own questions in order to get any information? *Should* I have any questions? If my doctor is not forthcoming with information and I don't know anything about the specific issues regarding my treatment, how am I supposed to know what I should be asking?

And whatever happened to patient-centered care and informed consent? Aren't patients supposed to understand what treatments they are receiving, the side effects/risks of such treatments, and so on? Why do I keep feeling that I don't know what they're doing to/with me? Why do I have to keep looking up medical journals and Internet sites to get information about my condition? Certainly, all my doctors have asked me to provide consent before they started any procedures. However, when obtaining consent, my doctors seem to care *only* about protecting themselves from liability; ensuring that I have a good understanding of what is going on doesn't seem to be a priority for them. They all seem to think of informed consent as a single event. Dr. Feber's staff, for example, asked me to sign an informed consent form when I came in for my first consultation meeting, and since then, I have received almost no new information regarding my treatment progress. It's as if these healthcare professionals think that when I signed and dated on the dotted lines a few weeks ago, they had fulfilled their obligation to obtain informed consent. Perhaps they think that they no longer have a duty to tell me anything else. However, it seems that, at least in cases where treatments are ongoing, doctors should keep checking in with their patients to make sure that they understand the progress of their treatment.

When I came in this morning, the therapists told me in an off-handed manner that they were changing my treatment. I asked them what that meant, and they said that I was going to enter "phase two" of my treatment. I didn't recall hearing anything about different phases at my original consultation a few weeks ago. When I tried to get a bit more information, they briefly noted that now they were going to treat the general breast area. I asked what that meant, and how that differed from phase one, and the therapists told me that Dr. Feber would explain it to me after the treatment. I wondered why they could not simply tell me a bit about phase two *prior* to starting this treatment, but since everyone seemed to be in such a hurry, I didn't want to hold anyone up. I knew that the next patient was already waiting outside.

So, when Dr. Feber asks if I have any questions today, I raise the issue. "How many phases are there to my radiation treatment? I knew I was getting radiation treatment for seven-and-a-half weeks, but I did not know that there were different phases to it. The therapists said I am now in phase two, and that they are treating the general area. Why did they change the treatment? Was it not working well before?"

If Dr. Feber is surprised that I am asking two-weeks-worth of questions in thirty seconds, she doesn't let it show. Without moving many muscles on her face, she quietly answers, "No. There was nothing wrong with the previous treatment. This change is a routine strategy. Usually after the first two weeks, we change the focus. We started with concentrating on the tumor site, but now we are treating the whole breast. This seems to be more effective for certain patients."

Certain patients. But not all of them? Am I one of the *certain* patients? And if it may be more effective, why didn't they start with that from the beginning? I ask Dr.

Feber all these questions, thinking that I should get some answers, especially if they're charging $483 every week for a consultation.

"Well," Dr. Feber hesitates. "It's kind of complicated to explain this." She pauses again.

I want to tell her that I am an intelligent person and that she can at least try to explain it to me. Besides, is it not the doctor's job to explain complicated matter in an understandable way to patients? It seems that effectively communicating complex but relevant or requested information to the patient is a challenge to which the doctor must rise. After all, despite the surge of medical websites and other academic resources, doctors continue to be our main source of information.

I push the matter hesitantly, realizing now that she might not have really wanted me to ask her any questions at the "consultation." She might have been hoping or expecting that I would simply tell her that I trust her judgment. "I'm just curious because I did not know that there would be any change in the treatment," I say apologetically, although I wonder why I should feel guilty about asking any question directly related to my care. "You mentioned that this change of treatment works well for *some* patients. What makes you think that this will work well for *me*?"

After a couple silent seconds, Dr. Feber finally gives me a simple answer. "It seems that the phase two treatment is not as effective for women with large breasts."

What is so complicated about that answer? Why didn't Dr. Feber simply tell me that when I first asked her about "phase two"? I am not asking for complicated statistics—I simply want to know why they changed my treatment.

Twenty years ago, Jay Katz wrote in *The Silent World of Doctor and Patient*[2] that the phrase "informed consent" is a deceptive slogan. It seems that his view still holds true today. Certainly, many healthcare professionals now recognize that respect for patients' autonomy is necessary to promote patients' self-determination and well being. However, it seems that many healthcare professionals still are not fully prepared to engage in meaningful conversations with their patients. Despite the increasing acceptance of patient autonomy, physicians continue to believe that they are the dominant members of the professional relationship, and many of them inadvertently make their patients silent agents in their association. Even though studies have shown that many patients prefer sharing decision-making with their physicians, many doctors still seem to control how much information they share with their patients. While Dr. Feber starts our weekly consultation by asking me if I have any questions, I have never felt that she wants to hear any response from me other than "no." When she tries to dismiss a question by saying that the information is "complicated," I feel like she is patronizing me. It is as if Dr. Feber only wants me to agree with her recommendations, follow the "routine," and not question her authority.

October 6, 2003

It has been almost eight weeks since I started my radiation treatment. I am quite excited that today is my last day of treatment! My skin has been burning and blistering a bit because of the radiation, so I am glad that this will be over soon. My scarred breast has turned dark brown, and I still have marker-lines and stickers all over my chest.

My medical experience has been humbling. As a bioethicist who often discusses issues of autonomy and physician-patient relationships, I have had little control over my own care. Despite my uneasiness with surgeries and radiation treatment, I have mostly followed my doctors' orders. Every time when I want to challenge their recommendations or request more information, I worry that they may be upset with me.

My experience with the radiation treatment has also forced me to redefine my identity and reconsider my body image. I did not put much emphasis on my external appearance prior to this experience. However, my treatment routine has made me a lot more conscientious about how I and others see my own body. Prior to my breast-cancer diagnosis and subsequent treatments, I thought that the main physical characteristic that distinguished me from most other women in this country was my skin color. While I was fully aware that we live in a society that is obsessed with breasts as sexual objects, I did not think that my breasts were a significant part of who I was or how I related to other people. I simply assumed that my breasts were part of a body that was *not* fragmented, *not* diseased, *not* unsexual. It was a body that was *mine*—I had control over it. However, my unpredicted diagnosis and the effects of my medical procedures forced me to renegotiate the very terms of my identity. For the last seven weeks, my diseased breast was under constant scrutiny by various therapists and doctors, who controlled every aspect of the treatment. My scarred breast became the center of attention—it framed my conversation with friends and family, and it also defined my therapeutic relationship with my healthcare providers. I would come into the radiation clinic every weekday and lie on the same treatment table as still as possible. They would move my arms and position me each day; it was as if I were a robot or a mannequin. I would watch the therapists measure my scar area, stare at the green lights that fragment my breast, and then go through the treatments. I would wait for them to finish the treatment and give me the "green light" to move and get dressed.

Thinking of my body as robotic and fragmented has helped me to try to desexualize myself in the treatment room and deal with the whole treatment process, but it has also caused pain in various ways. There is no changing room in the treatment area, but only a partially concealed corner with a small curtain that does not close completely. Maybe they think a changing room is unnecessary. After all, the therapists will be looking at my breast in a few minutes anyway. Nonetheless, having someone able to see me change in the room and then stare at my breast while I am on the treatment table has been embarrassing. And what's even more awkward is that I can't tell them not to stare! Something that is often considered taboo in our society has become a legitimate activity in my case. They all have received the license to stare, judge, and probe, because the breast is seen as a disjointed part of me—a diseased and dissected part that calls for investigation and damage control. It is a scarred part of my body, in the third-quarter of the breast, as the pathologist noted in my chart. My healthcare providers see my breast as a diseased part of my body, and I also start to think of it in similar ways. I no longer think of it as a sexual part of me, representing femininity or sensuality. Perhaps these healthcare professionals learn to forget about the social norm that dictates that breasts represent eroticism and sexuality and instead, are taught to think of the patients' breasts as simply clinical objects. And those gray hospital gowns with multiple strings are certainly not erotic lingerie. They match the dull colored walls of the radiation treatment room, such that one blends in with the surrounding and disappears in the impersonal area. Perhaps the ugly gowns are designed with the purpose of preventing any sexual feelings that doctors and other healthcare providers may have towards their patients. Or maybe they are designed to help the patients desexualize themselves so that patients feel comfortable having others measure, touch, and stare at their breasts as well as other parts of their bodies. If I thought my therapists were staring at me in a sexual manner when I was changing or while I was lying on the table with my bare-breasts, I probably would refuse to go through the treatments.

Yet, even if the healthcare providers have learned to desexualize the breast, can a patient, especially a young woman, be expected to do so? Especially when she is in the midst of a social culture that continues to measure a woman's worth and desirability by certain physical characteristics?

Prior to my diagnosis, I did not pay much attention to my breasts. While I realized that they represented a feminine and sexual side of me, I did not *want* to pay attention to them. However, I now start to worry that others may measure my worth and desirability by my breasts. More importantly, I worry that I myself may think in those terms. I wonder how other women with breast cancer feel about all this. Being the number one cancer among women, there are many articles and books about coping with breast cancer. However, they usually only focus on various medical options for treatment and not the psychological issues that breast cancer patients may face, especially those relating to sexuality. Some of them teach women how to keep a feisty attitude, while others discuss nutritional and exercise regimes. While many of these articles discuss reconstructive surgery options for patients who go through mastectomies, they are relatively quiet regarding body and sexual image. I am a bit puzzled that people don't discuss these issues widely, given our culture's obsession with breasts as sexual objects. Perhaps this is something that many people simply find too difficult or awkward to discuss. The fact that my mother "forgot" that two of her aunts had breast and ovarian cancers and her insistence that I should not tell anyone about my condition makes me feel that the diagnosis is something shameful, or that I am now a damaged body.

I find myself facing two opposing forces. On the one hand, I remind myself that I am not defined by my physical appearance and sex appeal—my intellectual ability and my relationships with my family and friends should count more. I try to tell myself that my identity as a person need not change because of my condition and surgeries. I remind myself that sexuality and femininity are both social constructs, and as a feminist who teaches at a women's college, I have an ethical responsibility to reject patriarchal standards of what it means to be a woman rather than succumb to various stereotypes of sexuality and gender that continue to oppress women around the world.

On the other hand, being situated in a culture that continues to hold various gender and sexual norms, one of my defense mechanisms involves convincing myself that I am still a sexual being, and that breast cancer and surgical scars do not take away my sexual desirability. Being a heterosexual woman who has not had children, I suddenly find myself trying to prove my womanhood. I worry about what my scars and cancer may do to my relationship with my partner. Although I have tried to convince myself that my lopsided and scarred breast does not change my inherent worth, the way that many of my friends stare at my chest area after I told them about my condition reminds me that even my most supportive friends cannot resist the breast culture.

It is ironic that I am unable to defy the culture that I try to convince my students to reject. I feel embarrassed that, at the moment of truth, I have succumbed to the breast culture. I sometimes stand in front of the mirror, trying to find ways to correct the lopsidedness of my breasts. I refuse to let Carl look at my scarred and burned breast, worrying that his desire for me will diminish. He tries to assure me that he still finds me attractive and desirable, but I doubt that he can escape the same breast culture that has somehow conquered me. Last night when I told Carl about my theory of heterosexual male therapists having to think of women's breasts as simply fragmented and diseased body parts in order to prevent inappropriate sexual thoughts from arising, he said, "Trust me. Breasts are breasts. Heterosexual men look at women's breasts as arousing, whether they are scarred or not!"

I don't know whether or not Carl is correct that heterosexual men find a burned and scarred breast, like mine, sexually arousing. But if he is, should I take this as another assuasive piece of "good news"? It seems that either way, I am trapped in the breast culture.

Anita Ho, Ph.D. is Associate Professor in Philosophy and Co-Coordinator of the Center for Women, Economic Justice, and Public Policy at the College of St. Catherine in St. Paul, Minnesota.

NOTES

1. All the names in this diary have been changed to protect the anonymity of all parties.

2. Jay Katz, *The Silent World of Doctor and Patient.* (New York: Free Press, 1984).

CHAPTER SIX

DEBRA GOLD

BREAST CANCER:

The Maternal Body Reflected in a Three-Way Mirror

"Please take a bath with me. Why won't you take a bath with me?" At first Lili's protestations are mild, even winsome. But over time my reluctance to shower or bathe with my five year-old daughter becomes irksome to her, then a source of rage and fury. "You have to take a bath with me or I won't take one. I can't take a bath alone." Her sense that she has lost an essential part of our relationship because of my mastectomy, the casual pleasure of being naked with mommy, the reassurance of our bare skins touching under the warm bath water, is not something she can put into words, but she can express her loss in her boycott of solitary bathing.

~

I remember loving my mother's breasts. They seemed enormous to me as a child, cascading onto her chest and her belly when she was nude, full and supple when corseted in the long-line bras and girdles she wore beneath her clothes. My mother used to call me into her room sometimes as she got dressed, and as we chatted I would examine her large breasts with curious eyes, comfortably, openly. Often, she would invite me to help her secure the hooks and eyes of these long brassieres around her fleshy back. It was a ritual I both cherished and feared. I wondered with excitement and a tad of dread what it would feel like to grow up and have to clad my own mountainous breasts in such tight undergarments.

When my mother had her first mastectomy, I was seven years old. From that time on, if she were undressed, she would call out from behind her locked bedroom door, "Wait a minute. I'm not dressed yet." I felt I had been abruptly banished from the Garden of Eden.

~

I enter Lili's room silently, to peek at her and Alexis playing, my presence unbeknownst to them. The outpouring from the imaginations of my six year old daughter and her friends delights me, their endlessly shifting identities as they

89

M.C. Rawlinson and S. Lundeen (eds.), *The Voice of Breast Cancer in Medicine and Bioethics,* 89-94.

parade about in bits of found cloth and ribbons, hats and oversized shoes dragged in from all corners of the house, as well as from the dress-up box we've assembled. Lili and Alexis are giggling. Lili has my two breast prostheses protruding from under her shirt, and my tired black wig is balancing precariously on her small head. Apparently she found a way into my closet. "Aren't I a woman?" she titters happily. "These are my mother's. She has cancer, you know."

~

I was never that uninhibited myself as a child, I don't recall ever even playing dress-up, except at Halloween, and then only to don the readymade costume my mother (when she was well) brought home from Woolworth's. I was, I think, too full of sadness, even then, and it kept me tied up, constricted, precociously solemn. My mother had breast cancer and I felt scared and small in the tumult around her illness. There were no corridors in my mind I could traverse to find respite.

~

I am having surgery yet again. Lili, at seven, sometimes mixes up words. "Are they going to put pimples on your breasts this time?" she wonders aloud. "Not pimples, sweetie, the doctor will be making nipples on my breasts," I reply. "Will I be able to drink milk out of the nipples?" she asks, half-joking, half-longing.

The next week, I look over and with pen in hand Lili is enhancing the drawings in her book about mermaids. "Do you see what I'm doing?" she asks, in a teasing tone. "Show me." Lili flips through her book to reveal the breasts and nipples she has given to each of the mermaids. Is she too obsessed, I wonder? How could she not be?

Lili has seen me naked now through several stages of surgery, before my cancer with my two natural breasts, then following a lumpectomy with one of those breasts severely scarred. Since I decided that being forbidden access to my naked body might be more traumatizing than the painful reality, Lili has seen me post-mastectomy with one breast only, and now, following a second mastectomy and double reconstruction, with two breasts, shapely mounds but one quite scarred and with no nipples. I have tried to explain the tram flap reconstruction I underwent in simple terms. But how is a child to make sense of all these changes in her mother's body, of the ways in which her mother's body has been transformed by illness and by science?

~

When my mother had her first mastectomy she was 38. It was 1962. There was no such thing as breast reconstruction. My mother lived with one breast through my childhood. When she had another episode of breast cancer requiring a second mastectomy at 64 it was 1989. Techniques of breast reconstruction had been developed by then, but my mother, who had been through so much hardship in her life, decided not to put herself through further "unnecessary" surgery.

My mother used to wear a breast prosthesis whenever she went out, and the prosthesis was a source of some angst. When my mother lost weight, she'd have to be re-fitted, and swimming required special bathing suits from a special store and different, waterproof prostheses that made her suitcase very heavy whenever we traveled somewhere warm. At home she could wear featherweight prostheses that fit into her specially prepared nightgowns or bathrobes. But at times my mother chose to relax around the house, and she would enter the living room in a robe through which I could make out the shape of just one breast, and one absent breast. This would fill me with despair and sometimes disgust, and I still feel guilty for the latter. (I try to forgive myself because now I know that the disgust was a thin mask I allowed myself to disguise my fear.)

~

"Don't lay on the couch, mommy. Once you lie down, you don't get up. Sit up, sit anywhere else." Lili was sick of seeing me reclining on the red Victorian sofa in our living room. I would sit down, thinking I was just going to rest for a minute, but then it was as though my leaden body was transfixed, and I would watch my family conducting their lives from a semi-slumber, some liminal space between wakefulness and sleep, life and death.

I had always been fond of sleep, but during chemotherapy discovered a level of tiredness I had never known was possible. Now I understood the phrase "bone tired." I felt my exhaustion in every cell. During the day I would rest on the couch to at least be near my family. Early in the evening, sometimes at six o'clock, sometimes eight, I would know that I needed to drop whatever I was doing and go to sleep instantly. Some of this may also have been because of depression. Sleep provided a brief reprieve from the terror and loss I was experiencing. My doctor proposed taking Dexedrine for energy, because she felt at points that my depression was related more to my loss of energy than to the illness itself.

~

My mother's body seemed to be molded to the large brown upholstered armchair by the living room window. She would sit there for hours, gazing out, her face drawn in grief, her eyes faraway. Only once, I saw her crying as I approached her from my bedroom, and it terrified me.

When my mother was ten her nineteen-year-old sister, Esther, died of bone cancer. The year my mother was diagnosed with her first episode of breast cancer, her twin sister, Ree, died of ovarian cancer. In the years ahead my mother's two remaining sisters, Sadie and Fay, also died from ovarian cancer. My mother dressed frequently in black dresses, with a small black ribbon pinned to her lapel to indicate she was in mourning. I would brush the white dandruff from her back and shoulders, and I would beg her to get a different dandruff shampoo so the white specks wouldn't show up on her dress. I finally got up the nerve to ask her to wear bright colors, but she didn't, not then.

~

Lili is preoccupied with physical appearance and thinness in a way I never was. I gained weight, about twenty-five pounds, through the course of my illness and treatment, and she started accusing me of being fat. (By objective standards I am not overweight, though certainly heavier than before.) I told Lili that I am not fat and that she could not insult me that way. Now she sometimes jokingly tells me I'm pretty but "flubbery." She relentlessly examines my face or body, depending upon accessibility, square inch by square inch, and she remarks on any new dot, line, or squiggle, or suddenly she notices and comments on a feature that's been present all along, such as a small birthmark on my left pinky. It exhausts me, this being under a microscope, and this being of infinite interest to my daughter. She can judge herself harshly as well, though at times she is quite admiring of her thinness (there is not an ounce of fat on her little body) or her hairstyle.

Lili is a very picky eater. She says she could eat more kinds of things but would have to hold her nose to do it! During chemotherapy I had no appetite, although between treatments I ate as though making up for lost time, and later I found it hard to lose that weight. I try to remember if Lili's appetite deteriorated when I was in chemotherapy. I wonder whether her pickiness is developmental and likely to pass or whether it could be a precursor to anorexia. I am a psychologist, and I can't help thinking about the theory that says many adolescent girls stop eating because they don't want to develop into women, they want to avoid developing curves and breasts.

~

After her first episode of cancer my mother gained a great deal of weight. She spent many years thereafter in a gain-lose-gain cycle, and the Weight Watchers food scale was part of our kitchen décor for years. My mother later explained to me that the problem was that whenever she lost weight she became anxious that it meant she had cancer again. Her weight was a kind of hedge against cancer, a safety barrier she had erected.

~

"Hold me like you would hold a baby." At seven, Lili still enjoys nothing as much as snuggling in her mother's or father's arms. During the course of my treatment I had to rely frequently on family and friends to pick up Lili from school, and she was often sent on play dates at her friends' houses, albeit sometimes reluctantly, so I could rest. Lili had her first sleepover when I needed to be in the hospital overnight after a twelve-hour surgery, and her father, aunt, and grandmother wanted to be with me until I came out safely from the recovery room. Her older brother was still too young to watch her. She slept at her best friend's house that night, and seemed to have a great time, notwithstanding her concerns about me. But at points during the treatment, and consistently once it slowed down, Lili insisted that I not leave her, she refused play dates at her friends' homes and would have them only at her own, and she repeatedly expressed her wish to be a baby again. Lili is left with a residue; call it uncertainty, insecurity, or anxiety. She keeps a close watch on me and insists that I keep one on her as well. And she wishes almost desperately that we could return to the time before my breast cancer complicated her childhood.

~

When I had my first chemotherapy treatment, I thought with irony about how I had always tried to eat healthy foods only, yet here I was with a needle in my arm injecting me with poison. I remember lying on the table for my first radiation treatment. I was filled with trepidation. All my life I had been led to believe radiation kills, yet here I was about to permit the technicians to blast me full of radiation. With each surgery, I dreaded not waking up from anesthesia, never seeing Lili and her brother again, not being here to raise them. At night I sometimes woke from deep sleep in a panic. When she asked, I tried to admit to Lili that I was scared at moments, but at the same time I did my best to be very positive, strong, hopeful, and reassuring. Children read their mother's true feelings. My breast cancer anxiety is in the air she breathes.

~

The windows of my second grade class looked out first to the schoolyard, then to my backyard and home. I would frequently sneak peeks out the window to see if I could catch glimpses of my mother in the garden, in the house, getting into the car. Then I looked out and tried to hold back my tears because she was gone. When she was in the hospital, Hilary (my older sister) and I walked home from school every day and stayed at Betty's house. She was my mother's best friend, and she was caring for us while our father was at work or visiting the hospital. Betty fed us tuna fish sandwiches. Our parents never made us eat tuna. We hated those sandwiches but never complained. For many years after, I gagged if I tried to eat tuna.

People didn't talk openly about cancer in those days. My father took me for a walk and told me that my mother was in the hospital because she had fallen and hurt her arm. In fact, my mother would come out of the hospital with bandages on her arm because she had a radical mastectomy that included removing all the lymph nodes. That was standard procedure then. My mother's arm swelled up immediately from lymph edema, and it never went back to its previous size and shape.

On Thanksgiving we visited my mother in the hospital. I was so relieved to see her, but I hated seeing her trapped in a hospital bed, attached to machines. She had always been vital and competent; in the hospital she seemed utterly weak and helpless. When she finally returned home, one of her no doubt well-intentioned friends instructed me that it would be my job from hereon in to be very well behaved and to take care of my mother. I felt, and was, much too little for such an enormous assignment. A housekeeper/babysitter came to live with us "just for awhile" to help out. I wanted my own mother to take care of me. Nothing was the same anymore. I was so scared. The burden of trying to be a good caretaker wore me down over the years that followed.

~

"I don't want you to read to me. Only daddy can read to me." Here came the flip side of Lili's profound attachment to me post-treatment. For a long time, I was so exhausted, so busy with medical appointments and therapies, so depressed by my illness and my fears of possibly dying. I had to depend on others and primarily on my husband to take over my parenting at a moment's notice. Whereas previously I had been the parent who read to Lili each night, he now read to her instead, as well as sharing many other special intimacies with her.

It was enormously difficult for me to agree to a mastectomy. I feared I would no longer be me without my breasts. When I discovered post-mastectomy that I felt, surprisingly, still myself, I also expected to be able to re-claim my prior life. But aside from the changes in me that made that precise life no longer possible or desirable, my family had moved ahead in ways I'd never foreseen, and I found I sometimes felt extraneous. They had learned of necessity to function without me and perhaps found it too dangerous to let me re-insert myself in the familiar ways. I still get hurt and angry with regard to this. It feels like a secondary injury on top of the cancer itself, a retaliatory abandonment that no one warned me about. In fact, I know it is not within Lili's conscious control and I will have to patiently re-gain her trust. Sometimes, now, she is like an infant angrily and helplessly beating her little fists against her mother's broken body.

~

My mother and I have discovered that we have the BRCA gene mutation that predisposes the women in certain families to develop breast and/or ovarian cancer. My mother torments herself about having passed this gene on to me, even though she and I both know with our rational minds that it was not her fault, that we are both equally innocent and equally hapless victims of this proverbial genetic roll of the dice. I want more than anything for my children to be spared such devastating illness in their lives, and also I want to survive to care for them should anything bad ever befall them, just as my extraordinarily courageous and nurturing mother has cared for me throughout my illness and treatment. I think with gratitude and relief about the fact that my husband and I adopted Lili when she was born. She is every bit our daughter, yet she is not our biological daughter. In this case that fact brings great relief. Though Lili and I may be quite alike in our childhood reactions to our mother's breast cancers, I do believe that the reflection of the maternal body in this three-generational mirror may finally have a chance to be transformed to one of good health.

Debra Gold, Ph.D. is a Clinical Psychologist and Psychoanalyst in private practice in Nyack, New York. She is a graduate of New York University's Postdoctoral Program in Psychoanalysis and she is a member of the Psychoanalytic Society of New York University. Dr. Gold is a former faculty member of the Albert Einstein College of Medicine, Department of Psychiatry.

CHAPTER SEVEN

LEATHA KENDRICK

LEARN TO LOVE WHAT'S LEFT

Poems on Breast Cancer

Second Opinion

We're four women waiting among a shifting set of others
in radiology's store-front lobby—three daughters
and a mother linked by blood and laughter
over *Cosmo Girl's* "most embarrassing
moments" (trail of toilet paper from the back of slacks,
the inevitable period started when you're wearing white,
a student asking her teacher, "If your quizzies are hard,
what about your testes?") Lyda loves that last one—
my funny last one—she's the performer, the mime.
Thank god, she's mine, feeding me one-liners.

The middle one, Eliza, brought my x-rays here,
and parked the car. She works the crossword,
all attention like her father but she's part of me,
my watching self. And Leslie, eldest, watches over us all,
rails against this three hour wait, tries to breach
the impersonal walls of disinterest in our fate. She was first
to nurse from this right breast, that pressed and prodded,
and later slicked with gel will echo sound onto a screen
to show the probable malignancy. I'm going to lose it—

the breast—and along with it the cancer, too, I hope.
The receptionist gives us a hard look when we laugh.
We're linked, silvery with a happiness
glinting out even in this waiting place.
I finger the necklace I've just bought, touch
the curative moonstone, murmuring "hope"—
I want to believe in sudden remission,
in some way to avert what we are certainly
headed for. What I can believe in
is the healing of their fingers laced through mine.

95

M.C. Rawlinson and S. Lundeen (eds.), *The Voice of Breast Cancer in Medicine and Bioethics*, 95-101.

Sonogram

The normal tissue flows by under her probe,
looking like grass under water. Her name is Laura—
a radiologist whose warm smile belies the hours
she's waited for me, both of us stuck in the slow
machinery of the appointment schedule. "Two lesions
near the nipple—between one and two o'clock"
she says. It's so quiet. I'm thinking,
"But it's nearly five!" Lame joke, left unspoken.

Instead I watch it on the screen, the sinuous
normal tissue, branching faintly white on gray.
I can almost feel it brush against my face
inside its dark. I want all my tissue to be like this,
but she's sounded me, slick of gel across
the veil of skin. She's found
these spiky shadows—ill-defined "masses,"

rocks in the stream. I see them too,
sharp yet indistinct, like something seen
through fog—a place to run aground, snags of log
and brush. I'm caught. She stayed long enough
to get the picture, the only clear one of the day.

The gel's cold and the gray threaded waver
of the screen take me to Aunt Ella's lake
where we tried the cold water and startled
at the weeds that clung and swirled
about our feet. Aunt Ella watched us,
arms across her chest in her large,
old-lady suit. "Breast cancer" was the
whisper hovering over her. And then
she was gone.

Christmas, Adolescence, Yin and Yang

My first love called them Skeeter and Bite.
Equal, then, if small. Skeeter got most
of his attention. Now that right
breast's shadowed, a dark harbor
to what will not differentiate, but does
its incessant adolescent dance. Light
and unseen shadow. Eye of light in darkness,
eye of darkness in light— two nipples
staring from one divided chest. They'll lift
one out, the eye sewn shut by mastectomy.

At this festive time of year, God's breast
sees all, bears all. His eyes never
shut. Mary suckled Jesus, and in some
theologies, the milk of human kindness
flows from His chest. At any rate,
that yearning to reach down and lift
someone to the heart does not depend
on breasts (I'm grateful to the man
who told me this, his eyes dark with grief.)

And yet, I lie abed touching the soft weight
splayed from breastbone to underarm and wonder
how we'd treat these dugs, these tits if God Herself
floated forever and ever Amen in Heaven above
with lovely heavy downward reaching breasts.

Costume. Fakery. The Sell:
On watching TV two weeks post-mastectomy

Excuse me while I grow bald and fat.

Sorry to offend the eye with my

one breast. I'm female. I apologize.

I fake two breasts, but know this half-flat

chest. I'll take chemo and a wig,

touch my losses secretly. No big

deal! I never have and never will

fit anyone's ideal. And I'm no star-

fish: won't regenerate. Fiberfill

and silicone help to hide the scar.

This new shape won't fill t-shirts, sell a car.

I'm served up on the half-shell. Turn off

the TV. Its cleavage shouts, "Are you buying?"

Avert your eyes. I've one soft side. I'm off

the market. Alive! Tender, I'm not hiding.

Pear Tree Mastectomy

This cutting winnows me
it prunes to harvest.
I am become a tree—
not Daphne's frozen flight
but a woman full,
in situ,

               and I will hope
to grasp any low branch, hold
on even as I let go of
what's not needed
any more,

               the scar riding
its bent branch up my chest
under my arm. I'm half-
mammaried. Too old
to play Peter Pan
or SuperMom,

               I'm gone
to seed, to see what's
next, what builds its
nest in this hollow space
where once I bloomed
white, milky, heavy
as a pear.

Learn To Love What's Left

Her breasts echo heaven's arc or
the Duomo with its nippled cupola—
two cathedrals, whose art is
irreplaceable. Instead of frescoes
one contains a Milky Way,
constellated calcified—a sectioned sky
with stars so thick she feels them
rising through the skin one July day—
as if Creation happened in the flash or brief week
physicists and the Bible say it did.

Some part of her inner universe has gone
supernova in a chain reaction
nothing (they say) can reverse.
It's blossomed, condensed
into two lesions (she imagines
deep space photographs,
explosions, petals with rayed edges
red and blue). Tongueless,
they can only reflect sound
onto a mute screen,
shadows in a threaded night.

Once the scalpels separate this starry dome,
this chapel, from her chest, nothing
makes it live again. That Universe, that Milky
Way is lost. The map back is a flat
red road, underpinned with bone,
she must learn to dance upon.

"Chance Favors the Prepared Mind"

The words uncoiling scare me now.

Then I could bear anything—all those months

I read every article on "locally advanced

survival," "combined modalities." Week after week

believing that Pasteur was right, knowing "chance

favors the prepared mind,"

I used my Apple to grasp my chances. I had to

listen to the coiled seducer caught in my right breast,

to leave the Garden of what you don't know

might well kill you. Meanwhile,

I took the drugs and lived

knowing no matter how well I prepared,

every doctor still dwelt in that place

before the accidental flash *past* the known,

where by grace or chance, some prepared mind

will comprehend the snake.

Leatha Kendrick holds an MFA in Poetry from Vermont College. She has taught creative writing for the University of Kentucky and Morehead State University. These poems are from a chapbook, Science in Your Own Back Yard, *published by Larkspur Press in 2003.*

CHAPTER EIGHT

GAIL WEISS

DEATH AND THE OTHER

Rethinking Authenticity

Death is a possibility of being that Da-sein always has to take upon itself. With death, Da-sein stands before itself in its ownmost potentiality-of-being. In this possibility, Da-sein is concerned about its being-in-the-world absolutely. Its death is the possibility of no-longer-being-able-to-be-there. When Da-sein is imminent to itself as this possibility, it is completely *thrown back upon its ownmost potentiality-of-being. Thus imminent to itself, all relations to other Da-sein are dissolved in it. This nonrelational ownmost potentiality is at the same time the most extreme one. As a potentiality of being, Da-sein is unable to bypass the possibility of death.*
——— *Martin Heidegger,*   Being and Time, *p.232*

Whether I was accepting my possible demise or denying it, I wanted very much to talk about it. I wanted to be keenly aware of what was happening to me, what death might mean, how it would feel. I didn't want to be cheated out of the experience because the subject was taboo. Or course, it was nearly impossible to discuss such an unknowable subject in any rational way. But I demanded that my family and friends engage me on this matter. And I'm happy to report that, to the last one, they have risen to the occasion.
——— *Cathy Hainer,*   The Cathy Hainer Journals, *p.29*

In Martin Heidegger's famous analysis of the existential phenomenon of being-toward-death in *Being and Time*, he emphasizes again and again that the radical "mineness" of death renders me incapable of authentically communicating anything about my own experience of its "indefinite certainty." Cathy Hainer, by contrast, suggests that one is "cheated out of the experience" of being-toward-death if one is unable to talk about it with others. The contrast between Heidegger's claim that death is Dasein's "ownmost *nonrelational* possibility" that "dissolves" our relations to all other human beings, and Hainer's "demand" that others can and must become actively engaged in the experience of her impending death, could not be more profound. What is at stake here is precisely the status of the other and, more specifically, our relations with others in the pursuit of what Heidegger terms "authenticity," or what we might term a meaningful and ethical life.[1]

M.C. Rawlinson and S. Lundeen (eds.), *The Voice of Breast Cancer in Medicine and Bioethics,* 103-116.

Cathy Hainer was not a philosopher like Martin Heidegger. She did not, to my knowledge, ever study phenomenology, but was a journalist for many years with the international newspaper, *USA TODAY*. Not only did Hainer share her own experience of "being-toward-death" with family and friends but also with millions of *USA TODAY* readers as she publicly chronicled her battle with breast cancer for eighteen months before she died in December of 1999. And the sharing continues after her death as I share her story with you.

One of the most important lessons that feminism has taught us is not to seek wisdom only through established channels. That is, just as feminists have sought to recover the lost wisdom of those whose voices were never heard while they were alive because they lacked the proper gender, proper race, proper sexuality, proper class, and proper education to have their knowledge recognized and affirmed, so too, we must continue to question false boundaries that artificially divide different forms of inquiry—including those that separate formal philosophies from more informal (but no less rigorous) discussions of the very meaning of human existence. Despite the criticisms of phenomenology that have been raised over the years by feminists and others who argue that its descriptions of lived experience are very limited insofar as they are utterly dependent on the perspective of the one who is providing them, I would argue that phenomenology is uniquely suited to the feminist political project of recognizing the legitimacy of the experiences of those people, such as Cathy Hainer, who lack the formal credentials to be recognized as "experts" in the interpretation of those experiences. Before I can make this case, let me acknowledge the force of the accusations against phenomenology as it has traditionally and officially been practiced.

Not only have phenomenological descriptions been viewed as suspect because of their alleged subjectivism, but they are also condemned because of the phenomenologist's sleight of hand in presenting his (invariably, and significantly it is a man's) own experience as the experience of all.[2] Paraphrasing Luce Irigaray's objections to Merleau-Ponty's phenomenology in particular, Elizabeth Grosz succinctly articulates Irigaray's central concern as follows:

> [For Merleau-Ponty] the world remains isomorphic with the subject, existing in a complementary relation of reversibility. The perceiving, seeing, touching subject remains a subject with a proprietorial relation to the visible, the tactile: he stands over and above while remaining also within his world, recognizing the object and the (sexed) other as versions or inversions of himself, reverse three-dimensional "mirrors," posing all the dangers of mirror identifications. (Grosz 1994, 107)

While Merleau-Ponty's anti-Cartesian understanding of the "body-subject" as being of the same "flesh" as the world it inhabits would seem to make him less guilty of subjectivism than other phenomenologists such as Husserl and Sartre who affirm the transcendence of the subject via the transcendence of human consciousness, the implication is that if Merleau-Ponty is guilty as charged, then all other phenomenologists and phenomenology itself are also discredited. The force and persuasiveness of this often-invoked criticism of phenomenology has led to something of an impasse for contemporary feminist phenomenologists. Not only are many of us eager to divorce ourselves from the unsavory reputation of being "subjectivists" but we must also defend our own commitment to phenomenology by showing that we do not intend to falsely universalize our own experience by portraying it as the experience of all.

There are many ways to engage in this latter project, and one of them, the one that I will pursue here, involves relaxing the relatively stringent criteria that determine who is and is not a philosopher, who is and is not a phenomenologist. This can be accomplished by recognizing the prevalence and power of phenomenological descriptions of experience that we find all around us especially those that are offered to us in what may seem to be the most unlikely of places, including the pages of *USA TODAY*, a media realm that seems to be an archetypical example of what Heidegger saw as the inauthentic domain of "the they." To be open, in advance, to the possibility that an authentic description of "being-toward-death" can come from an allegedly inauthentic venue, is to acknowledge that there is no one privileged site or mode of being that alone can reveal the most meaningful aspects of human experience.

I began by setting forth an antinomy between two views of being-toward-death, one offered by a professional philosopher in the course of a classic work of the twentieth century, *Being and Time*, and the other offered by a professional journalist in the course of a series of newspaper articles that detailed her terminal illness with cancer. How, one might ask, can Cathy Hainer's personal testimony of the importance of sharing her experience with others possibly challenge the authority and veracity of Martin Heidegger's proclamation that death dissolves my relations with all others by forcing me to confront on my own my "ownmost nonrelational possibility"? Doesn't her very attempt to share her experience, especially to share it in such an anonymous public forum as the media, condemn her from the outset to inauthenticity? Doesn't the radical "mineness" of death, a quality which I agree with Heidegger is one of its most crucial features, preclude the possibility of communicating anything about it to anyone else except insofar as we seek to avoid the anxiety of acknowledging that it is not only others but myself who is dying? Moving once again beyond phenomenology proper, I believe that it is in literature, namely in the pronouncement of Leo Tolstoy's Ivan Ilych that we can best see what is at stake in this terrible recognition:

> The syllogism he had learned from Kiesewetter's logic- "Caius is a man, men are mortal, therefore Caius is mortal"- had always seemed to him correct as applied to Caius, but by no means to himself. That man Caius represented man in the abstract, and so the reasoning was perfectly sound; but he was not Caius, not an abstract man; he had always been a creature quite, quite distinct from all the others. (Tolstoy 1981, 93)

And Ivan continues, "Caius really was mortal, and it was only right that he should die, but for him, Vanya, Ivan Ilych, with all his thoughts and feelings, it was something else again. And it simply was not possible that he should have to die. That would be too terrible" (ibid., 93-94).

In the transition from the true premise that all human beings are mortal to its necessary and equally true conclusion that as a human being "I, too, will die," Ivan experiences the tremendous anxiety of having his relations to all other Dasein undone. Indeed, Ivan's continual wavering between an authentic awareness that his death is imminent and cannot be avoided, and an inauthentic denial that this could really be true for him, offers an incredibly strong example of the power of the they to "tranquillize" individuals about their own (and others') deaths. As one who has lived his own life by conforming to the they's understanding of what is "pleasant and proper," Ivan cannot find any resources within the they to confront the unpleasantness and impropriety of his illness and impending death. Indeed,

> He saw that the awesome, terrifying act of his dying had been degraded by those about him to the level of a chance unpleasantness, a bit of unseemly behavior (they reacted to him as they would to a man who emitted a foul odor on entering a drawing room); that it had been degraded by that very "propriety" to which he had devoted his entire life. (Tolstoy 1981, 103)

Over time, Ivan comes with great difficulty and much suffering to recognize that while his inability to resume his position as an active participant in the public domain of everyday life sets him apart from others, it also provides him with a unique and hitherto unlooked for opportunity to interrogate his own existence on its own terms, apart from the dictates of the they. In his solitary meditations on his own being-toward-death, Ivan affirms Heidegger's assertion that:

> Death is the *ownmost* possibility of Da-sein. Being toward it discloses to Da-sein its *ownmost* potentiality-of-being in which it is concerned about the being of Da-sein absolutely. Here the fact can become evident to Da-sein that in the eminent possibility of itself it is torn away from the they, that is, anticipation can always already have torn itself away from the they. The understanding of this "ability," however, first reveals its factical lostness in the everydayness of the they-self. (Heidegger 1996, 243)

As a result of his previous "lostness in the everydayness of the they-self," Ivan finds himself poorly equipped to confront the limitations of the knowledge provided to him by the they head-on. "[W]hy should I have to die, and die in agony?" he asks.

> Something must be wrong. Perhaps I did not live as I should have," it suddenly occurred to him. But how could that be when I did everything one is supposed to?" he replied and *immediately dismissed the one solution to the whole enigma of life and death, considering it utterly impossible.* (Tolstoy 1981, 120; emphasis added)

In this pivotal passage in the text, Tolstoy shifts swiftly and almost imperceptibly from the first person account of Ivan's questioning of his experience to the narrator's observation that in Ivan's rejection of the idea that he may have lived inappropriately even though he faithfully followed the dictates of the they on how to live appropriately, he at the same time "dismissed the one solution to the whole enigma of life and death." Paradoxically, Tolstoy reverts to the voice of the anonymous narrator to convey a truth about Ivan's own experience that is, at the time, no more than a nightmarish possibility to Ivan himself, a possibility that he hastily repudiates, namely, that the socially acceptable life he has hitherto led has been inauthentic precisely because it is society (and not Ivan) who has dictated the very terms through which that life has been given meaning and value.

Although Ivan Ilych seems like a perfect example of Heidegger's call to throw off the shackles of the they when confronting our own being-toward-death— precisely because the they, with its constant and myriad forms of tranquillization about death can never provide us with the resources to deal with it on a personal, immediate level—Tolstoy also challenges Heidegger's picture of Dasein resolutely facing its death cut off from all others in his description of the final moments of Ivan Ilych's life. As he acknowledges without flinching that the entire way in which he has lived his life, that is, in accordance with social convention, has been the wrong way to live, Ivan suddenly is freed from his former resentment and even hatred toward his wife and all those others who are still able to live life in accordance with the they and for whom his pain and suffering has been an unseemly and incredibly difficult burden to bear. Even while recognizing that his wife, daughter, former colleagues, and the doctors will resume their habitual activities without giving his death more than a passing thought, Ivan also recognizes that his suffering has tortured them and that he must forgive them for not also confronting the inadequacy of the they which has served them so well:

> And suddenly it became clear to him that what had been oppressing him and would not leave him suddenly was vanishing all at once—from two sides, ten sides, all sides. He felt sorry for them, he had to do something to keep from hurting them. To deliver them and himself from this suffering. "How good and how simple!" he thought. (Tolstoy 1981, 133)

Despite the fact that Ivan is too weak to communicate these feelings of love and regret to his family, Tolstoy depicts him as at peace because "He who needed to understand would understand" (Tolstoy 1981, 133). In his sudden discovery of God's presence (a presence that has not manifested itself until this point), Ivan is able to forgive himself and forgive others for their previously inauthentic relations by entering into an authentic relationship with God. Unlike Tolstoy, however, Heidegger does not hold out the hope that God will provide an authentic alternative to the inauthenticity of the they. For Heidegger, one cannot appeal to any transcendent being to give one peace in reckoning with one's own being-in-the-world without also condemning oneself to inauthenticity yet again precisely because God is, by definition, not of this world.

Albert Camus describes this appeal to the religious in order to escape the absurdity of an existence that lacks any source of external justification as a primary example of "the spirit of nostalgia" (Camus 1991, 42) and he excoriates it even more vigorously than Heidegger who simply identifies it as a common strategy employed by the they to diminish Dasein's anxiety toward death.[3] Despite the power of Heidegger's and Camus' respective rejections of any appeal to God to alleviate one's suffering in confronting one's being-toward-death, and despite the artificiality in which God suddenly appears to "save" Ivan from the they at the end of Tolstoy's story, one may still question whether Heidegger and Camus have not reacted too hastily in seeing any reaching out to others (or to God) as attempts to mediate that which cannot be mediated, namely a personal confrontation with one's own mortality.

In *The Stranger*, Camus's Meursault, on the eve of his death by the guillotine, rejects and even mocks Ivan Ilych's divine vision of the possibility for human love and forgiveness in the very presence of the priest who comes against Meursault's will to administer the last rites:

> Actually, I was sure of myself, sure about everything, far surer than he; sure of my present life and of the death that was coming. That, no doubt, was all I had; but at least that certainty was something I could get my teeth into—just as it had got its teeth into me. I'd been right, I was still right, I was always right. I'd passed my life in a certain way, and I might have passed it in a different way, if I'd felt like it. I'd acted thus, and I hadn't acted otherwise; I hadn't done *x*, whereas I had done *y* or *z*. And what did that mean? That, all the time, I'd been waiting for this present moment, for that dawn, tomorrow's or another day's, which was to justify me. Nothing, nothing had the least importance, and I knew quite well why. He, too, knew why. From the dark horizon of my future, a sort of slow, persistent breeze had been blowing toward me, all my life long, from the years that were to come. And on its way that breeze had leveled out all the ideas that people tried to foist on me in the equally unreal years I then was living through. What difference could they make to me, the deaths of others, or a mother's love, or his God; or the way a man decides to live, the fate he thinks he chooses, since one and the same fate was bound to "choose" not only me but thousands of millions of privileged people who, like him, called themselves my brothers. (Camus 1954, 151-152)

Camus goes one step further than Heidegger, in fact, by rejecting the very possibility of authenticity insofar as it connotes the possibility of giving meaning to one's existence (even on one's own terms). For Camus, there is no meaning at all, just absurdity. Or, one might say, the meaning of human existence *is* its absurdity. He acknowledges the human demand for meaning and justification but also proclaims that it will never be met.

How might the following entry from Cathy Hainer's journal be squared with such a bleak vision?

> And I can't help imagining what my own obituary will say: "Cathy Hainer graduated from college and went to work for a newspaper." Will I be disappointed that it doesn't describe me as "Pulitzer Prize winner and author of best-selling novels"? A little. But I hope I'm more concerned with my legacy than my obituary. Will people remember me fondly? Have I brought a smile to anyone's face, helped anyone out of a difficult time? Have I made someone laugh when they were down, done anything for the common good of mankind? (Hainer 1998-99, 34; Hainer 1999a)

Whereas the "deaths of others, or a mother's love or his God" or even the love of his girlfriend Marie are of no concern to Camus' Meursault, Cathy worries about how she will be remembered. She is not concerned with recognition of her professional accomplishments but with the effects, both small and large, that she hopes to have had on the lives of others. As Cathy anticipates her death, contemplating the transformation of its indefinite certainty to a definite one, she receives her greatest pleasures from the affection and love she gives and receives with her family and friends:

> Saturday mornings can be a hectic time at my house, but a few weekends ago we actually were able to lounge late in bed. David [Cathy's fiancé] was dozing peacefully on one side of me, and Maggie, my adorable new dachshund puppy, was curled up in

the crook of my other arm. For me, that was nirvana. I feel a little sheepish having such
ungrandiose dreams, but my friend Anne says that's the sign of a life well lived. I hope
she's right. (Hainer 1998-1999, 30; Hainer 1999b).

It is clear that the peace and happiness Cathy feels with loved ones by her side
does not eviscerate the anxiety she experiences knowing that her cancer and bodily
discomfort will get much worse and that it will end up killing her. She does not
evade this realization in the journal but she does share the intimacy of this personal
journey with family, friends, and millions of strangers. From a Heideggerian
perspective, as we have seen, the radical individualization of death separates me
from all others, undoing my relationship with other Dasein and presumably with
animals such as Cathy's dog Maggie. To attempt to share the experience, he
suggests, is a form of inauthentic flight that distorts its very essence as mine. It is
important to note that in the example above, Cathy is sharing her experience silently,
through the warmth of her body as it embraces the warmth of David's and Maggie's
bodies. Here, there is an intercorporeal exchange taking place, simply through the
communication between bodies. Would Heidegger view this nonverbal exchange as
inauthentic as well? And, why should words render a relationship inauthentic to
begin with?

In the following passage, Heidegger reiterates but then seems to retreat from the
strong claim that Dasein can no longer have any relations at all with others when it
is authentically confronting its ownmost possibility, namely, death:

> The nonrelational character of death understood in anticipation individualizes Da-sein
> down to itself. This individualizing is a way in which the "there" is disclosed for
> existence. *It reveals the fact that any being-together-with what is taken care of and any
> being-with the others fails when one's ownmost potentiality of being is at stake.* Da-sein
> can *authentically* be *itself* only when it makes that possible of its own accord. But if
> taking care of things and being concerned fail us, this does not, however, mean at all
> that these modes of Da-sein have been cut off from its authentic being a self. As
> essential structures of the constitution of Da-sein they also belong to the condition of
> the possibility of existence in general. Da-sein is authentically itself only if it projects
> itself, *as* being-together with things taken care of and concernful being-with...,
> primarily upon its ownmost potentiality-of-being, rather than upon the possibility of the
> they-self. Anticipation of its nonrelational possibility forces the being that anticipates
> into the possibility of taking over its ownmost being of its own accord. (Heidegger
> 1996, 243; emphasis added)

We can understand Dasein's failure to take care of things when confronting
authentically its being-toward-death as a failure to express its previous level of
concern for its everyday projects, just as Ivan Ilych failed to take the same pleasure
in card playing, working, and decorating his house that he had before. However,
when Heidegger says that there is also a failure to be concerned more generally, this
suggests that Dasein no longer experiences the same sense of care for its own
existence. The question becomes, is the failure to be concerned a failure in our very
ability to care? But care is the very structure of Dasein's being for Heidegger, so if
our ability to care is at stake then Dasein's own being as Dasein is also at stake.
Perhaps for this very reason, Heidegger goes on to suggest that even though there is
a failure to take care of things and a failure of concern when one confronts one's

impending death authentically, these "modes of Dasein" haven't been cut off completely since they are the very "condition of the possibility of existence in general."

As existential structures, then, taking care of things and being concerned are still part of our very make-up as Dasein and so they remain structures of our being, Heidegger implies, even as they suffer failure. But the question I am interested in here is not the formal persistence of these existential structures but their content or lack thereof. For, if the structures remain, but are empty, then how much can they really be contributing to the meaningfulness of my existence? Is there any existentielle content that we can give to these structures and to the relationships that flow (or fail to flow) from them without falling into inauthenticity? What, precisely, is the status of Dasein's concrete, everyday relations with others and with the world of its concern—relations which Heidegger has claimed are dissolved when Dasein confronts its *ownmost* potentiality that cannot be outstripped?

In the quote above, Heidegger attempts to negotiate this tension by distinguishing between grounding these relationships upon the they-self, an inauthentic move, versus "the possibility of taking over its ownmost being of its own accord." On a generous reading, we may say that Dasein is able to live its relationships authentically in its being-toward-death so long as it grasps these relations on its own terms rather than society's. Fair enough. But what about the terms of the other, terms which are not reducible to my own but which also play a key role in my relations with that other? There seems to be no room for any other perspective here.

Defending Heidegger against the charge that an authentic life can only be lived solipsistically, Tina Chanter asserts that "Dasein's self-understanding is structured by its tendency to derive its meaning from its meaningful relations with the world" (Chanter 2001, 80). If this is so, she suggests, then relations with others can and should play a valuable role in Dasein's authentic relationship to its own being-toward-death, especially since others are included in that being as it is lived out ontically. The problem, both she and I agree, is that Heidegger's own account seems to preclude this because of his failure to distinguish the inauthentic public domain of the they sufficiently from an authentic way of being-with-others in the form of a community. While Heidegger does emphasize the importance of social and political traditions in establishing Dasein's own historicity, he also laments Dasein's tendency to become *ensnared* in those traditions, depriving itself of its own voice and perspective:

> Da-sein not only has the inclination to be entangled in the world in which it is and to interpret itself in terms of that world by its reflected light; at the same time Da-sein is also entangled in a tradition which it more or less explicitly grasps. This tradition deprives Da-sein of its own leadership in questioning and choosing. This is especially true of *that* understanding (and its possible development) which is rooted in the most proper being of Da-sein—the ontological understanding. (Heidegger 1996, 18-19)

Pulling Dasein away from its "proper" ontological understanding of its being, Heidegger suggests, is not only tradition but our own they-self. "In being-toward-death" he tells us:

> Da-sein is related to *itself* as an eminent potentiality-of-being. But the self of everydayness is the they which is constituted in public interpretedness which expresses itself in idle talk. Thus, idle talk must make manifest in what way everyday Da-sein interprets its being-toward-death. (Heidegger 1996, 233-234)

How are we to distinguish between our inauthentic they-self and our authentic self on this account? Ultimately, Heidegger see-saws back and forth on whether or not our relations to others and the world of our concern are necessary casualties along the path of authenticity. What is clear is that he can give no content to such relations and that his own views must cause us to view loving descriptions of those relations, such as those provided by Cathy Hainer, with suspicion.

Tina Chanter turns to Emmanuel Levinas for a more satisfactory account of the essential role played by the other in our being-toward-death. Indeed, for Levinas, Death is the Other, pure alterity, violent and beyond comprehension. "The violence of death" he tells us,

> threatens as a tyranny, as though proceeding from a foreign will. The order of necessity that is carried out in death is not like an implacable law of determinism governing a totality, but is rather like the alienation of my will by the Other. It is, of course, not a question of inserting death into a primitive (or developed) religious system that would explain it; but it is a question of showing, behind the threat it brings against the will, its reference to an interpersonal order whose signification it does not annihilate. (Levinas 1969, 234)

Death, on Levinas' account, cannot take us away from the other but leads us straight toward the other; death is yet another, but most special, instance of the ineradicable transcendence of the other in relationship to me.

But Cathy Hainer's descriptions of her relations with others in the months before her death focus not on the radical alterity of the other(s) but on the intimate ways in which she and they are able to *traverse* the distance between them, enriching their respective lives in the process. The fact that Cathy's personal narrative of this process also had an impact on millions of people she never met makes it extremely problematic for both Heidegger and Levinas. Undoubtedly, Cathy had a *relationship* with her readers, one that she nurtured in the final months of her life in full awareness of the power of her narrative to trigger a personal response from them. Such a relationship seems to typify the very meaning of the they-self on Heidegger's account, after all what could be a more effective use of public interpretedness than the media? However, what I am arguing here, is that Cathy Hainer's clear-eyed phenomenological description of her being-toward-death provides evidence of the limitations of Heidegger's account not only of being-toward-death and the role of the they, but also of authenticity itself.

In the months following the September 11, 2001 terrorist attacks in the United States, *The New York Times* published a series of biographical sketches every day in which family members and friends provided interviewers with brief descriptions of the life of a particular victim. These "profiles of grief" tended to emphasize the mundane aspects of each individual's existence including where these people lived and how they got to work each day, the names of their partners, children, and pets, the food they best liked to eat, the places they most liked to travel, and the things in life they valued most.[4] One of the reasons the accounts have been so moving, I believe, is because *in* the very mundanity of the life being described, something unique about each life is simultaneously communicated. The paradoxical ability to reveal the unique in the typical and familiar, I would argue, is precisely what must be done justice to if we are to make sense of the relationship between death and the other. Rather than encountering an ineffable alterity on the one hand or the inauthenticity of the they-self on the other, Hainer's narrative and these profiles remind us of the alternatives in between, alternatives that both challenge and reconfigure our very notions of subjectivity and alterity, death and authenticity.

One alternative to solipsistic conceptions of subjectivity is provided by Kelly Oliver in her recent work on witnessing. According to Oliver,

> addressability and response-ability are the conditions for subjectivity. The subject is the result of a response to an address from another and the possibility of addressing itself to another. This notion of subjectivity begins to go beyond the categories of subject, other, and object that work within scenarios of dominance and subordination. (Oliver 2000, 41)

Despite the promise of such a relational account of subjectivity, Oliver ends up embracing a Levinasian vision of our relationship to others, insofar as the other itself is depicted as being beyond our comprehension:

> To recognize others requires acknowledging that their experiences are real even though they may be incomprehensible to us; this means we must recognize that not everything that is real is recognizable to us. Acknowledging the realness of another's life is not judging its worth [Taylor], or conferring respecting [*sic*], or understanding or recognizing it, but responding in a way that affirms response-ability or addressability. We are obligated to respond to what is beyond our comprehension, beyond recognition. Ethics is possible only beyond recognition. (Ibid., 41-2)

While it is certainly true that I cannot be said to comprehend the other in his or her entirety without vanquishing that very otherness, and while it is clear that cognitive comprehension of the other would give us only a very partial view of who that other really is, I would argue that an *existential* comprehension of the other *as* other is possible and that it can be made even more meaningful precisely when we come face to face with our own mortality.

In opposition to what I take to be a false dichotomy between the absolute alterity of the other on the one hand, and the complete knowability of the other on the other hand, my point is that we do not need to embrace the incomprehensibility of the other in order to do justice to the other's alterity. Although I agree that my comprehension of the other will always exceed the capacity of conventional discourse to represent it, I am also maintaining that it is conventional discourse that continually points us toward it. Thus, conventional discourse, as we have seen through the examples of Cathy Hainer's journals and Tolstoy's story of Ivan Ilych, *can*, contra Heidegger, lead us toward authentic experiences of ourselves in relation to the other and to our own death, experiences that *can* and indeed *must* be expressed and communicated through the language of the they.[5]

Moreover, these experiences, even when enacted through discourse, inevitably possess, as Maurice Merleau-Ponty has shown us, a corporeal and, more precisely, intercorporeal dimension. That is, the response-ability and addressability discussed by Oliver always involves our bodies which are called to respond to the bodies of others.

The intercorporeal exchanges between bodies issue, I would argue, from what I have elsewhere called a series of "bodily imperatives" that demand them.[6] That these relationships can be inauthentic or authentic is undoubtedly true, but their authenticity must be determined not by rejecting their mundanity, but in and through it.

Gail Weiss is Associate Professor of Philosophy and Director of the Graduate Program in Human Sciences at George Washington University.

NOTES

1. I do not intend to suggest here that meaningfulness and ethicality together are synonymous with authenticity for Heidegger. Authenticity is a very complex, rich notion in his work and cannot be done justice to through the notions of meaningfulness and ethicality. However, I do think that it is impossible to achieve any measure of authenticity in one's life if meaningfulness and ethicality are not present.

2. There have been so many of these criticisms directed against so many major figures in the phenomenological tradition (including Heidegger, Sartre, Merleau-Ponty, Levinas, and Beauvoir) that they cannot all be mentioned here. Contemporary continental feminist theorists who have raised them include: Luce Irigaray, Julia Kristeva, Judith Butler, Elizabeth Grosz, Iris Young, Sonia Kruks, Kelly Oliver, Tina Chanter, Debra Bergoffen, Dorothea Olkowski, and Shannon Sullivan—and these are only the tip of the iceberg!

3. Turning to God, an "otherworldly being," for comfort in dealing with the angst of one's own being-toward-death would seem to be, for Heidegger, yet another way in which the they seeks tranquillization about death. In his words, "The this-worldly, ontological interpretation of death comes before any ontic, other-worldly speculation" (Heidegger 1996, 230).

4. See nytimes.com/portraits for the complete group of biographical sketches that have been created to date. *The New York Times* has also published these portraits as a book. The most recent edition is, *Portraits: 9/11/01: The Collected "Portraits of Grief" from* The New York Times, *Revised Edition* (New York: Times Books, 2003).

5. I believe that this position is closer to Judith Butler's than to Kristeva's or Irigaray's. For, Butler rejects the possibility of preserving a separate domain of language, such as Kristeva's semiotic or Irigaray's maternal-feminine, from the symbolic order and she is suspicious of claims that escape from the symbolic is necessary in order to subvert hegemonic interpretations of the subject and its others. What I am saying is that we need not escape conventional discourse in order to express truths about human existence that are unique and personal. See Butler's, "The Body Politics of Julia Kristeva," *Hypatia* 3, no. 3 (1989): 104-117 for her detailed critique and response to the appeal to pre-symbolic experience as a way of getting beyond the limitations of the symbolic domain.

6.   See chapter 7 of my *Body Images: Embodiment as Intercorporeality* (1999) for a description of
     bodily imperatives and their foundational role in motivating an embodied ethics.

REFERENCES

Beauvoir, Simone de. 1989. *The Second Sex*. Tr. H.M. Parshley. New York: Vintage Books. (Orig. pub.
     1949.)

Bergoffen, Debra. 1997. *The Philosophy of Simone de Beauvoir: Gendered Phenomenologies, Erotic
     Generosities*. Albany: State University of New York Press.

Butler, Judith. 1993. *Bodies that Matter: On the Discursive Limits of Sex."*   New York: Routledge.

——— 1990. *Gender Trouble: Feminism and the Subversion of Identity*. New York: Routledge.

——— 1989a. Sexual ideology and phenomenological description: A feminist critique of Merleau-
     Ponty's *Phenomenology of Perception*. In *The Thinking Muse: Feminism and Modern French
     Philosophy*, eds. Jeffner Allen and Iris Marion Young, 85-100. Bloomington: Indiana University
     Press.

——— 1989b. The body politics of Julia Kristeva. *Hypatia: A Journal of Feminist Philosophy* 3, no. 3:
     104-117.

Camus, Albert. 1991. *The Myth of Sisyphus and Other Essays*. Tr. Justin O'Brien. New York: Vintage
     Books. (Orig. pub. 1942.)

——— 1954. *The Stranger*. Tr. Stuart Gilbert. New York: Vintage Books. (Orig. pub. 1942.)

Chanter, Tina. 2001. *Time, Death, and the Feminine: Levinas with Heidegger*. Stanford: Stanford
     University Press.

——— 1995. *Ethics of Eros: Irigaray's Rewriting of the Philosophers*. New York: Routledge.

Grosz, Elizabeth. 1994. Volatile Bodies: Toward a Corporeal Feminism. Bloomington: Indiana
     University Press.

——— 1993. Merleau-Ponty and Irigaray in the flesh. *Thesis Eleven* 36: 37-59.

Hainer, Cathy. 1999a. A lesson learned outside the lab: To keep living. *USA TODAY*, July 19: D7.

——— 1999b. Learning to live after cancer comes back: A clean bill of health then "a bomb" in brain
     and body. *USA TODAY*, April 20: D1.

——— 1998-1999. *The Cathy Hainer Journals. USA TODAY*. (The original articles appeared between
     March 10, 1998 and December 6, 1999 in the "Life" section of *USA TODAY*). These articles are
     available through the *USA TODAY* electronic archives at www.usatoday.com.

Heidegger, Martin. 1996. *Being and Time*. Tr. Joan Stambaugh. Albany: State University of New York
     Press. (Orig. pub. 1927.)

Husserl, Edmund. 1970. *The Crisis of European Sciences and Transcendental Phenomenology*. Tr. David
     Carr. Evanston: Northwestern University Press. (Orig. pub. 1954.)

——— 1962. *Ideas: General Introduction to Pure Phenomenology*. Tr. W.R. Boyce Gibson. New York:
     Collier Books. (Orig. pub. 1913.)

Irigaray, Luce. 1993. *An Ethics of Sexual Difference*. Tr. Carolyn Burke and Gillian C. Gill. Ithaca: Cornell University Press. (Orig. pub. 1984.)

———— 1985a. *This Sex Which is Not One*. Tr. Catherine Porter. Ithaca: Cornell University Press. (Orig. pub. 1977.)

———— 1985b. *Speculum of the Other Woman*. Tr. Gillian C. Gill. Ithaca: Cornell University Press. (Orig. pub. 1974.)

Kristeva, Julia. 1982. *Powers of Horror: An Essay on Abjection* . Tr. Leon S. Roudiez. New York: Columbia University Press. (Orig. pub. 1980.)

———— 1980. *Desire in Language: A Semiotic Approach to Literature and Art*. Ed. Leon S. Roudiez, tr. Thomas Gora, Alice Jardine, and Leon S. Roudiez. New York: Columbia University Press. (Orig. pub. 1977.)

Kruks, Sonia. 2001. *Retrieving Experience: Subjectivity and Recognition in Feminist Politics*. Ithaca: Cornell University Press.

———— 1990. *Situation and Human Existence: Freedom, Subjectivity and Society* . London: Unwin Hyman.

Levinas, Emmanuel. 1969. *Totality and Infinity: An Essay on Exteriority*. Tr. Alphonso Lingis. Pittsburgh: Duquesne University Press. (Orig. pub. 1961.)

Merleau-Ponty, Maurice. 1968. *The Visible and the Invisible* . Ed. Claude Lefort, tr. Alphonso Lingis. Evanston: Northwestern University Press. (Orig. pub. 1964.)

———— 1962. *Phenomenology of Perception*. Tr. Colin Smith. London: Routledge & Kegan Paul. (Orig. pub. 1945.)

The New York Times. 2003. *Portraits: 9/11/01: The Collected Portraits of Grief from*   The New York Times, *Revised Edition*. New York: Times Books.

Oliver, Kelly. 2001. *Witnessing: Beyond Recognition*. Minneapolis: The University of Minnesota Press.

———— 2000. Beyond recognition: Witnessing ethics. *Philosophy Today* 44 (Spring): 31-42.

Olkowski, Dorothea E. 2000. The end of phenomenology: Bergson's interval in Irigaray. *Hypatia: A Journal of Feminist Philosophy* 15, no. 3: 73-91.

———— 1999a. *Gilles Deleuze and the Ruin of Representation*. California: University of California Press.

———— 1999b. Phenomenology and feminism. In *Edinburgh Encyclopedia of Continental Philosophy*, 323-332. Edinburgh: Edinburgh University Press.

Sartre, Jean-Paul. 1943. *Being and Nothingness*. Tr. Hazel E. Barnes. New York: Washington Square Press.

Sullivan, Shannon. 2001. *Living Across and Through Skins: Transactional Bodies, Pragmatism, and Feminism*. Bloomington: Indiana University Press.

Tolstoy, Leo. 1981. *The Death of Ivan Ilych*. Tr. Lynn Solotaroff. New York: Bantam Books. (Orig. pub. 1886.)

Weiss, Gail. 1999. *Body Images: Embodiment as Intercorporeality*. New York: Routledge.

Young, Iris M. 1997. *Intersecting Voices: Dilemmas of Gender, Political Philosophy, and Policy* . Princeton: Princeton University Press.

———— 1990. *Throwing Like a Girl and Other Essays in Feminist Philosophy and Social Theory*. Bloomington: Indiana University Press.

III. BREAST CANCER AS A MODEL IN CLINICAL RESEARCH

CHAPTER NINE

JOHN S. KOVACH, M.D.

BREAST CANCER RESEARCH

A Political Cause and Paradigm for Scientific Inquiry

Breast cancer has been a focal point for passionate discussion by the public, the press, politicians, scientists and ethicists for the past fifty years.[*] Breast cancer is the leading cancer in women and breast cancer advocacy has swept the nation. Many private foundations, companies, communities, and schools have joined the federal government in funding breast cancer research and creating breast cancer awareness programs throughout the country. Due to recent advances in technology, we are now at the threshold of being able to discover the causes of cancer and implement strategies for its prevention. Technology has already brought us remarkable new tools for improving rates of early diagnosis and for estimating prognosis. If the public, politicians and scientists can find a way to partner in prioritizing projects and resources, there is an unprecedented opportunity to reduce the burden of life-threatening chronic diseases.

In many ways the saga of breast cancer detection and management is illustrative of sociopolitical forces which have driven the rise of women in the professional workplace and an increased openness about health and sexuality not imagined by the bobby soxers of the 50's, let alone their parents. After President Nixon's declaration of a War on Cancer in 1971, the concept of medical research as a military assault against disease became commonplace. There are advantages and disadvantages to such imagery. The advantage is that the call to arms mobilizes human and financial resources to engage an enemy that is terrorizing the nation. The great disadvantage is an expectation of a rapid and total victory when the odds overwhelmingly favor a protracted expensive struggle. The failure of scientists to inform politicians and the

---

[*] One student's response to Dr. Kovach's chapter is included in chapter 14 of this volume, pp. 203-207. The student, Sofya Maslyanskaya, participated in a conference on breast cancer at Stony Brook University where Dr. Kovach delivered an earlier version of this essay.

M.C. Rawlinson and S. Lundeen (eds.), *The Voice of Breast Cancer in Medicine and Bioethics,* 119-131.

public about the primitive state of knowledge of the complex nature of [breast] cancer allowed unrealistic optimism to sustain a strategy designed to conquer a simpler, more vulnerable enemy. Only recently has it become clear that cancers of a particular tissue are a spectrum of disorders ranging from benign to dangerous.

Barron Lerner recounts the last 100 years of breast cancer treatment in the United States in his outstanding history, The Breast Cancer Wars[1] (Lerner 2001). For most of the twentieth century breast cancer was not much discussed in society. It was an affliction to be borne in silence. When a lump was detected, a general surgeon, almost always male, performed an operation he felt appropriate based on his "clinical experience." Usually no therapy in addition to surgery was offered. At the beginning of the twentieth century, William Halsted, at Johns Hopkins University, seeing that many women with local and regional recurrence of breast cancer after varying types of surgery went on to die of widespread disease, decided that the best chance for cure was to remove the affected breast and as much adjacent tissue as possible. He pioneered a radical operation for primary breast cancer in which all soft tissue from the chest and under the arm was removed. This left a parchment-like covering of the ribs through which the expanding lungs were readily appreciated. Besides creating a dreadful cosmetic result, the radical mastectomy often resulted in marked swelling of the arm due to removal of the axillary lymphatic system. The swollen arm was a cause of embarrassment, generally painful, and a site of frequent and sometimes serious infections. Despite these complications, the radical mastectomy became the treatment of choice for all breast cancers. Halsted's influence was enormous and his approach to breast cancer was adopted by an entire generation of surgeons. To the credit of these technically gifted surgeons, there was an increase in breast cancer survival, although prospective randomized trials were not done to prove the point. Still, no more than 60% of women were cured with this approach.

The motivation behind the radical operation was to remove all cancer. It was dogma that, if any disease were left, a fatal outcome was inevitable. A few confident surgeons, working from institutional platforms that could provide security in the face of professional criticism, raised the possibility that a lesser operation might be as effective as the Halsted procedure. George "Barney" Crile, Jr. at the Cleveland Clinic was one of the few challengers, advocating in the 1950's a lesser operation and indeed had his first wife's breast cancer treated by a simple mastectomy (removal of the breast only) in 1961. His pioneering efforts helped bring about a slow but progressive reduction in the magnitude of surgery for breast cancer.

Subsequently a number of surgeons, in particular, Bernard Fisher at the University of Pittsburgh, spearheaded a series of landmark randomized studies of lesser operations for the management of breast cancer. These comparative trials showed that survival for ten years after treatment was about the same for radical mastectomy, simple mastectomy, and simple local excision of the cancer (lumpectomy), the latter accompanied by radiation to reduce local recurrence in the preserved breast. Studies done over 30 years culminated in the widely popular current approach of local removal of the cancer followed by six weeks of external beam radiation to the breast. Sampling of the first lymph node under the arm, expected to be involved if the cancer has already spread, is routine. If cancer is found, the other nodes are removed and/or irradiated. Chemotherapy, when given to high-risk patients based on lymph node involvement, further reduces the likelihood and time to recurrence in some women and is even recommended without lymph node involvement for a small potential benefit. An advantage for lumpectomy is a greater possibility for cosmetically acceptable breast reconstruction without major plastic surgery. A disadvantage of lumpectomy is that it must be followed by six weeks of x-ray to reduce the rate of local recurrence in the breast to 10% or less, the rate achieved with simple mastectomy alone (Abeloff et al. 2000).

At the beginning of the twenty-first century, the overall cure rate of breast cancer in the United States is greater than 80%. This is a significant improvement with much less extensive surgery compared to the days of Halsted. But the survival rate is a long way from the total victory expected when the war on cancer was declared and it took about 50 years to make this modest advance against the enemy. The absence of an accurate measure of the risk of fatal spread of breast cancer at the time of detection of a "lump," a problem recognized and emphasized early on by Crile and others, continues to preclude individualization of treatment.

In 2002, there were over 220,000 new cases and 40,000 deaths from breast cancer in the United States (American Cancer Society's Cancer Facts & Figures 2003). Virtually every woman is aware of these frightening statistics. The gradual success of women in bringing attention to the disease and facilitating an improvement in treatment established a powerful lobby. Women began asking why their families and those of many of their friends and neighbors seem plagued by breast cancer. Advocates began demanding more studies of the causes of the disease and of methods for early diagnosis while medical science continues its painstaking search for more effective less toxic treatments. The breast cancer war proceeds in the twenty-first century in local and regional battles often marked by frustration, anger, and disappointment at the slow pace of progress. "Why can we put a 'man' on the moon yet fail to conquer the most common cancer of women?" is commonly asked at advocacy meetings.

In the 1980s, breast cancer advocates, particularly those in the Northeast, became convinced that environmental factors must play a role in the high incidence the disease in their region. Their ongoing battle for national attention on this issue is dramatically illustrated by the furious interplay of the press, politicians and the public over "targeted" funding for breast cancer research. Long Island advocates had long been concerned that the water supply and toxic waste sites on the island were causes of high rates of breast cancer. Advocates used their energies and prominence as voters to demand that legislators pay more attention to environmental toxins. Energetic volunteer organizations with names such as "Breast Help" and "One in Nine" on Long Island, joined forces with state and federal representatives to obtain funding for studying environmental causes of breast cancer and facilitating breast cancer screening. Breast cancer advocates had had stunning success nationally in lobbying Congress to create within the Department of Defense a mechanism for reviewing and funding breast cancer. (Since 1991, the United States Army Material Command has awarded over $1 billion for breast cancer research. See the Department of Defense website). The advocates on Long Island had a more modest success when Congress in 1993 directed the National Cancer Institute to support research on breast cancer in Long Island women.

Thirty million dollars were allocated to support 12 studies that became known as the Long Island Breast Cancer Study Project (LIBCSP). Among the studies conducted by several leading academic medical centers in New York State were evaluations of electromagnetic radiation from power lines and other sources in the home, polycyclic aromatic hydrocarbons, PAHs (combustion products of fossil fuels and tobacco) and pesticides (DDT and its breakdown products) as breast cancer carcinogens, development of a map of toxic waste sites throughout Long Island (which could eventually be overlaid with the location of the residences of breast cancer patients), and methods for improving rates of breast cancer screening.[2] Experts in epidemiology and environmental toxicology at academic institutions, the National Cancer Institute, and the National Institute of Environmental Health Sciences helped plan the research. A decision was made to study PAHs because these compounds were known to cause breast cancer in rodents (PAHs are also known to cause lung and bladder cancer in men) and because the organochlorine pesticides have female sex hormone-like activity and are widely distributed in the environment.

The first results of two of the twelve studies which investigated possible associations of PAHs (Gammon et al. 2002a) and of pesticides (Gammon et al. 2002b) with breast cancer were published in August 2002. The results did not indicate a significant association with either class of these ubiquitous environmental contaminants. There followed in the press, most notably *Newsday*, the largest daily paper on Long Island, a series of three articles highly critical of the two studies and the LIBCSP in general. The articles under the headline, "Tattered Hopes," were accompanied by an illustration of a pink ribbon, the symbol of breast cancer advocacy, in shreds.[3]

The articles included comments from scientists with distinguished titles in academia and the government, boldly stating, some nine years after implementation of the research, that it was obvious from the beginning that these studies were doomed to fail. The chief complaint of the press was that the country had been boondoggled out of $30 million by the raw political power of busloads of vociferous advocates backed by the then incumbent Senator Alphonse D'Amato. This alliance, it was complained, forced the federal government into providing money sufficient to mollify the constituents of Nassau and Suffolk Counties and preserve political power.

The following week, *The New York Times* ran a commentary by one of its distinguished science writers entitled "Epidemic that Wasn't"[4] in which the complaints elaborated at length in *Newsday* were echoed, leaving the impression that money had been wasted searching for an environmental cause of breast cancer. The major objection was that the advocates had overstated the magnitude of breast cancer incidence on Long Island, claiming it to be the highest in the country. A few days later, the editorial page of *The New York Times* piled on with "Breast Cancer Mythology on Long Island."[5] In this brief piece, a new thought was highlighted, namely that all-in-all there is probably no basis for believing that environmental factors are involved in breast cancer causation on Long Island and even if they were, it would not be possible to identify them.

What about the claims of *Newsday* and *The New York Times* of the use of political power to fund frivolous research? The use of political power to influence funding for a matter of broad public concern is not particularly shocking in New York politics. Congress does distribute some pork. The fact that a few sausages were directed toward a major concern of the public in a highly populated region was not disturbing to most.

What about the research? Careful study of over 1,500 women with breast cancer compared to 1,500 women without cancer failed to reveal a strong association between PAHs or organochlorines and the disease. The data did raise the possibility, however, that there are differences, at least in women, in the body's ability to eliminate PAHs. The well-characterized database and stored blood samples created by this study are being used for evaluating this possibility and will be available to explore new hypotheses as knowledge of the biology of breast cancer expands.

And it appears that the advocates' intuition about PAHs, at least those in cigarette smoke, was right on target. Very recently, a group of Canadian investigators showed that early smoking in pre-menopausal women who have never been pregnant and heavy smoking by women who have borne children significantly increases breast cancer risk (Band et al. 2002). Because the time of life at which one is exposed to potential cancer causing agents may be critical to cancer causation, the study of toxins in individuals who already have cancer may not reveal an association. For example, the only women in Hiroshima and Nagasaki who suffered increased rates of breast cancer were exposed to radiation as girls (Goodman et al. 1997).

The major objections to the motivation and strategies used by the advocates is that they overstated the risk of breast cancer on Long Island to gain their day in Congress and that it is unlikely that there are (identifiable) environmental causes of breast cancer. The latter is a serious issue because taken at face value there would seem to be little reason to push for discovery of preventable causes of breast cancer. Although reproductive factors (age of menarche, number of births, and duration of breast-feeding) are important factors in determining risk, it is widely acknowledged that environment and lifestyle are major contributors to the breast cancer epidemic in the West. Perhaps the strongest evidence is that when Asians migrate to the United States, within 10 years their rate of breast cancer almost doubles and the rate of their daughters and granddaughters rises to the extraordinary rates characterizing the U.S. population (Key, Verkasalo, and Banks 2001; Ziegler et al. 2001; Lacey, Devesa, and Brinton 2002).

North America has among the highest rates of breast cancer in the world similar to New Zealand, Northern and Western Europe. Rates are somewhat lower in the temperate regions of South America and still lower in Southern and Eastern Europe and the tropical regions of South America. The lowest are in Asia at levels 5 to 7 fold lower than in North America (Lacey, Devesa, and Brinton 2002). Where does Long Island fit in? Suffolk County is virtually tied for the third highest rate of breast cancer in the United States with Atlanta, San Francisco, and San Jose. The coastal neighbor of Long Island, Connecticut, just across Long Island Sound, is number two; and the leader, by a slim margin, is another coastal region, Seattle/Puget Sound. Thus, Long Island does have an extraordinary incidence of the disease. And because of its population of over three million, Long Island is a prime region to study the causes of breast cancer.[6]

The abrupt dismissal by the press of the results of the first two reports of the LIBCSP created disappointment and enhanced frustration among breast cancer advocates and raised suspicion that the war was not going well. This suspicion was boosted by a recent controversy over the value of mammography. A provocative analysis by Danish epidemiologists suggested that mammography did not result in any increase in breast cancer survival (Olsen and Gøtzsche 2001). A panel convened by the National Cancer Institute reviewed the data and agreed with the conclusion. The American Cancer Society challenged the interpretation stating that the value of mammography had been proven already and women should continue annual mammograms, certainly, from age 50 and for women at high risk, from age 40 (American Cancer Society's Cancer Facts and Figures 2003). About the same time, *The New York Times* ran a three part series pointing out the variable quality in mammography instrumentation and in the competence of radiologists interpreting mammograms.[7] These in-depth expositions about the technology accompanied by photographs of challenging mammograms alerted the public to the fact that even under the best circumstances, mammography is a helpful but rather imprecise tool. To the dismay of many, these reports were followed by a large carefully done study of the value of breast self-examination on improving breast cancer survival. Thousands of women in Shanghai were given repeated instruction and encouragement to do monthly self-breast examination. However, this group, while detecting more abnormalities in the breast including more breast cancers than an untrained comparable group of women, did not have improved rates of cure or survival (Thomas et al. 2002).

Each of these issues got wide coverage on national television, usually a 45 second spot implying that something is amiss in medicine or science at the public's expense. So, although women have overcome medical prejudice about the management of breast cancer and have helped improve the cure rate, it would seem to many in 2002, that we are no further along in understanding the causes of high rates of the disease in specific groups of women and that the mantra of early detection by self exam and frequent mammography is suspect.

The breast cancer battles waged for over a century continue today primarily because the enemy is still poorly understood and, therefore, difficult to engage in meaningful battle. The confounding feature of "breast cancer" (and many other cancers that look the same to the pathologist) is that it is not a single disease.

Discussions and research on causation, management, and risk have focused on an entity expected to behave similarly in all individuals. It has been obvious that some breast cancers, even when discovered as very small lesions, are destined to spread regardless of the treatment. Until recently, science has lacked the tools needed to reveal the complexity and capability of the enemy.

The measures for judging breast cancer are crude. These are: age, the number of axillary lymph nodes at the time of surgery, the size of the primary lesion, the appearance of the cancer cells on microscopic examination, and the presence or absence of molecular markers indicating the likelihood of growth dependence upon the hormones estrogen and progesterone. The later hormone receptor assays are widely touted and almost universally used in guiding initial treatment, yet offer little in the way of additional prognostic information over whether or not the cancer has spread to the lymph nodes.

However, recent technical advances and understanding of the regulation of cell growth hold the promise of dramatically improving methods of diagnosis and estimating prognosis for breast and other cancers. These opportunities stem from the recognition that all cancers and indeed, probably all non-infectious chronic diseases, result from altered genes (Hanahan and Weinberg 2001). A single cell in a particular tissue, like the breast, acquires genetic damage from a few genes that either puts the cell into overdrive or damages the brakes that control growth. The genetic alterations in the cancer are not present in other cells of the body. These gene changes can be caused by many agents including internal factors like oxygen products from the combustion of food and environmental factors such as tobacco and fossil fuel smoke, ultraviolet radiation, x-radiation, cosmic rays and many other naturally occurring and industrially produced chemicals. Fortunately, cells have remarkably efficient systems for repairing rapidly and accurately thousands of gene injuries cells sustain every day. And, since it takes damage to several specific genes to result in cancer, the odds are greatly against these rare events happening to just the right genes in the same cell.

The defense systems can be overwhelmed, however, by prolonged exposure to toxins as is the case for lung cells of chronic cigarette smokers and the skin of farmers which is bathed in ultraviolet radiation year in and year out. Also, some unlucky individuals are born with defective defense systems. Such persons develop cancer after levels of exposure to toxins that would not harm those with normal defenses.

A landmark scientific achievement of the past century was deciphering the details of the human genetic code (Venter et al. 2001; International Human Genome Sequencing Consortium 2001). The aggregate of all genes of a particular species, known as the genome, is the set of instructions for development from one cell to an independent functioning organism. When the instructions are incorrect, cells make incorrect products or regulate processes incorrectly so that abnormalities we recognize as disease may result. Deciphering the human genome has revolutionized the ability to study inborn and acquired (metabolic and environmental) risks of disease. Within the decade, it is likely that the entire genetic profile of an individual can be obtained at an affordable price and in a reasonable period of time, the "one thousand dollar genome in a day." (Sequencing of the first genome took ten years and cost three billion dollars). Given the pace of computational technology development, it will be possible to detect rapidly all gene differences between diseased and normal tissue in an individual and between individuals at high and low risk of developing specific diseases. Comparative genetic analyses will revolutionize medicine by indicating which gene variations are responsible for undue risk of specific diseases and provide targets for development of treatments tailored to exploit variations specific to the disease. Genetic analyses will also allow determination of whether the genetic alterations in diseased cells came about because of inborn or acquired (environmental) factors.

Indeed, the nature of the biochemical changes in acquired gene damage may implicate a specific class of environmental toxins as likely causes of disease. For example, the pattern of gene damage in lung cancers of cigarette smokers is highly suggestive of the effects of the toxins (PAHs) in cigarette smoke and is markedly different from the pattern of damage in the same gene in lung cancers of non-smokers (Hollstein et al. 1996). Fully 95% of lung cancers occur in smokers because of years of exposure to these toxins.

There is also strong circumstantial molecular genetic evidence indicating that environmental factors contribute to breast cancer development and that these factors differ in geographically different populations (Hartmann et al. 1997). Knowledge of patterns of biochemical damage in genes known to be associated with specific cancers should be of help in exploring the causes of the large differences in cancer incidence among different ethnic groups. Patterns of gene damage may also provide clues as to whether a "cancer cluster," an unexpectedly high rate of a specific type of cancer in a defined geographic region, is the result of a dominant toxin in the environment rather than chance alone.

"Hot spots" of breast cancer are reported from time to time. One of the most intriguing recent findings is that thousands of Caucasian women living in Marin County, California between the ages of 45 and 64 had an estimated 8% annual increase in breast cancer incidence from 1991 to 1997 (Clarke, Glaser, and West 2002; Prehn et al. 2002). There was no change in the incidence of breast cancer in younger or older women in Marin County and no increase in the disease at any age in the four neighboring San Francisco counties. There is no explanation for this "cancer cluster" as yet but known risk factors related to reproduction appear not to be the cause.

To illustrate the potential power of molecular epidemiology to shed light of the causes of such a cluster, let us hypothesize that many women in Marin County decided on the basis of reports of "mad cow disease" from Europe to take up a new diet. Assume they switched to fish as their main source of protein. Some of the most popular fish are among the most expensive. These would be affordable on a regular basis by an affluent family but not the average household.[8] Large fish, at the top of the food chain in the sea, are reported to concentrate in their tissues a variety of toxins such as PAHs, DDT and its breakdown products, mercury and other industrial chemicals (Davis, May, and Greenfield 2002; Harvard Health Letter 2003). If the above scenario were true, higher amounts of toxins in the new diet of affluent women in Marin County might increase gene damage that, in turn, increases the incidence of breast cancer. Comparison of patterns of gene changes in the cancers of the affected age group in Marin County to the patterns of gene changes in cancers of women from the surrounding counties might show biochemical differences compatible with greater exposure to specific types of environmental toxins in the higher risk group. Older affluent women may not have been as quick to make a big change in diet and younger women, even having embraced the new diet may not yet have been exposed long enough to have increased risk.

A "molecular epidemiological" approach to the study of cancer clusters is not usually possible because of the absence of detailed clinical and epidemiological data and frozen tissue samples essential for molecular analysis to say nothing of the cost. However, as technology becomes cheaper and pathologists routinely preserve tissue specimens not needed for diagnosis in a manner suitable for genetic and protein analyses, it will be possible to gain at least circumstantial evidence as to whether an environmental toxin or class of toxins play a dominant role in specific cancer clusters. Unfortunately, such analyses, even if negative, would not exclude the possibility that environmental factors are at play. For example, chemicals with hormone-like activity could increase breast cancer incidence by stimulating growth of cells, just as excess exposure to estrogen does, without leaving a distinctive pattern of gene damage.

It will be some time before comparative molecular genetic analyses becomes more widely used for detecting environmental causes of disease. However, molecular characterization of several cancers has demonstrated that we are on the brink of stunning improvements in estimating prognosis and early disease detection.

A recent study of breast cancer in women from the Netherlands is a good example of what to expect in the near future. Investigators working with Merck Pharmaceutical Company analyzed patterns of utilization of genetic information in breast cancers from women followed for ten years after diagnosis. The analytic technique, called micro-array, measures simultaneously the "expression" of thousands of genes. The investigators first measured expression of 15,000 genes in each of 50 breast cancers, which had been frozen at the time of surgery. Using computational techniques, they correlated the degree of gene expression with occurrence or lack of occurrence of cancer and found that patterns of expression of as few as 70 genes predicted prognosis (van 't Veer et al. 2002). They then applied their assay to 295 patients younger than 53 years of age with stages I and II breast cancer. They found a striking difference in the overall 10-year survival of about 55 % and 94% for patients with "bad prognosis patterns" compared to those with "good prognosis patterns," respectively (van de Vijver et al. 2002). The fact that certain gene changes may profoundly affect prognosis is not without precedent. Sommer and colleagues demonstrated that the presence or absence of a mutation in a single gene, the P53 gene, which is frequently altered in many different types of cancer, is also a better guide to estimating prognosis of breast cancer patients than any currently used clinical parameters (Kovach et al. 1996; Blaszyk et al. 2000; Hill and Sommer 2002).

Another truly extraordinary advance in cancer diagnosis, based on a different but complementary type of molecular technology, also has the potential to dramatically improve cure rates of cancers that commonly spread before causing symptoms. A consortium of investigators from the National Cancer Institute, the Food and Drug Administration, and a bioinformatics company, Correlogics, Inc. in Bethesda, Maryland, recently reported a simple rapid and, potentially low cost, blood test for the diagnosis of ovarian cancer (Petricoin et al. 2002a). The technology involves the science of "proteomics." Proteomics is the study of the structure and function of all proteins coded for by our genes. Each gene codes for one or more protein depending on how the information of the gene is used. Since proteins are a direct representation of the detailed sequence of the genes, alterations in gene sequence frequently result in the production of proteins with modified structure in lesser or greater amounts than in the "normal" individual. Using mass spectroscopy, an analytical tool that can measure accurately minute quantities of thousands of molecules and a mathematical tool for detecting unique features in a sea of virtually identical molecules, the investigators found a distinctive pattern of molecules in the blood of women with ovarian cancer. In a blinded study, this assay detected all 50 of 50 blood samples from women with ovarian cancer and only miscalled 3 of 66 samples from individuals without cancer (Petricoin et al. 2002a). These scientists and others have extended proteomic analysis of the blood to the diagnosis of prostate (Petricoin et al. 2002b) and breast cancer (Li et al. 2002) with impressive results but without the same degree of specificity and sensitivity obtained for ovarian cancer.

The availability of a rapid inexpensive blood test that accurately predicts the presence of specific types of cancer at early stages will revolutionize the practice of oncology. For example, the current overall cure rate for ovarian cancer is a dismal 30% to 40% because the disease causes few symptoms until it is relatively advanced. Early diagnosis is certain to save many lives because Stage I ovarian cancer is known to be curable in more than 90% of patients. Whether the cure rate of breast cancer would increase significantly if an accurate blood test were available is not as clear cut, but the cost saving of substituting a blood test for mammography as the primary screening tool for breast cancer would be enormous and many more women would be willing and able to participate in screening programs.

In addition to the extraordinary benefit a blood test for early diagnosis of cancer would be to healthcare, if the cancer markers in the blood are the products of the altered genes of the underlying cancers, identification of these markers will lead directly to identification of the corresponding genes. The search for genetic damage leading to cancer could then focus on the culprits responsible for cancer development among the some 35,000 gene possibilities.

Somewhat surprisingly, none of the exciting studies discussed above have had the independent confirmation needed to bring them to clinical practice. This is true for many intriguing molecular studies of different cancers that are beginning to flood the medical literature. Even though the tools and knowledge are available to determine the causes and biologic behavior of chronic diseases like cancer, such research requires access to well characterized clinical data and properly preserved blood and tissue.

In his recent book, *Science, Truth, and Democracy* (2001), Philip Kitcher makes a compelling argument for striving toward a state of "well-ordered science" as we go forward in the twenty-first century. He addresses the great challenges facing science in deciding how to utilize the information from the human genome project and attendant technologies for maximum public benefit and minimum public damage. To accomplish this goal, Kitcher points out that there must be procedures for decision making which have the best chance of achieving a plan that meets the "collective wishes" of society. He sees the critical decisions as resource allocation, most efficient study design within ethical boundaries, and determining how results may be of practical benefit (Kitcher 2001).

Modern medical research depends on the public to play an intimate and complex role in the process, since the public is the subject, sponsor, and intended beneficiary. Scientists are appropriately proud of recent accomplishments and are eager to improve public health through a deeper understanding of disease. However, sustained funding for medical research will depend increasingly upon society's demands on government that such research have potential benefit for public health. Scientists must find ways to partner with the public so that these demands are appropriate and realistic.

NOTES

1. A few of the highlights of the tortuous saga of breast cancer management are described below but the reader is highly recommended to the carefully annotated fascinating account of Professor Lerner.

2. The web site for the LIBCSP, http://epi.grants.cancer.gov/LIBCSP/ details the history and lists each of the projects and participants of the LIBSCP.

3. *Newsday*, July 28, 29 and 30, 2002.

4. *The New York Times*, August 29, 2002.

5. *The New York Times*, August 31, 2002.

6. Annual age adjusted rates for 1994-98 from the National Cancer Institute and the New York State Department of Health as reported in "Tattered Hopes," *Newsday*, July 28, 2002. See also, www.newsday.com/health/ny.

7. "Blurred Vision," a three part series, *The New York Times*, October 22-24, 2002.

8. "Rich Folks Eating Fish Feed On Mercury Too," *San Francisco Chronicle*, November 5, 2002.

REFERENCES

Abeloff, M.D., J.O. Armitage, A.S. Lichter, J.E. Niederhuber, L.J. Pierce, and R.R. Love. 2000. Breast. In *Clinical Oncology, Second Edition,* ed. M.D. Abeloff, J.O. Armitage, A.S. Lichter, and Niederhuber, 2093-2094. New York: Churchill Livingstone.

American Cancer Society's *Cancer Facts and Figures*, 2003. http://www.cancer.org.

Band, P. R., N.D. Le, R. Fang, and M. Deschamps. 2002. Carcinogenic and endocrine disrupting effects of cigarette smoke and risk of breast cancer. *Lancet* 360: 1044-9.

Blaszyk, H., A. Hartmann, J.M. Cunningham, D. Schaid, L.E. Wold, J.S. Kovach, and S.S. Sommer. 2000. A prospective trial of midwest breast cancer patients: A P53 gene mutation is the most important predictor of adverse outcome. *International Journal of Cancer* 89: 32-38.

Clarke, C.A., S.L. Glaser, and D.W. West. 2002. Breast cancer incidence and mortality trends in an affluent population: Marin County, California, USA, 1990-1999. *Breast Cancer Research* 4: R13.

Department of Defense, *Congressionally Directed Medical Research Programs.* http://cdmrp.army.mil/bcrp.

Davis, J.A., M.D. May, and B.K. Greenfield. 2002. Contaminant concentrations in sport fish from San Francisco Bay 1997. *Mar Pollut Bull* 44: 1117-29.

Gammon, M.D., R.M.Santella, A.I. Neugut, S.M. Eng, S.L. Teitelbaum, A. Paykin, B. Levin, M.B. Terry, T.L. Young, L.W. Wang, Q. Wang, J.A. Britton, M.S. Wolff, S.D. Stellman, M. Hatch, G.C. Kabat, R. Senie, G. Garbowski, C. Maffeo, P. Montalvan, G. Berkowitz, M. Kemeny, M. Citron, F. Schnabel, A. Schuss, S. Hajdu, and V. Vinceguerra. 2002a. Environmental toxins and breast cancer on Long Island I: Polycyclic aromatic hydrocarbon DNA adducts. *Cancer Epidemiol. Biomarkers Prev.* 11: 677-685.

Gammon, M. D., M.S. Wolff, A.I. Neugut, S.M. Eng, S.L. Teitelbaum, J.A. Britton, M.B. Terry, B. Levin, S.D. Stellman, G.C. Kabat, M. Hatch, R. Senie, G. Berkowitz, H.L. Bradlow, G. Garbowski, C. Maffeo, P. Montalvan, M. Kemeny, M.Citron, F. Schnabel, A. Schuss, S. Hajdu, V. Vinceguerra, N. Niguidula, K. Ireland, and R.M. Santella. 2002b. Environmental toxins and breast cancer on Long Island II: Organochlorine compound levels in blood. *Cancer Epidemiol. Biomarkers Prev.* 11: 686-697.

Goodman, M.T., J.B. Cologne, H. Moriwaki, M. Vaeth, and K. Mabuch. 1997. Risk factors for primary breast cancer in Japan: 8-year follow-up of atomic bomb survivors. *Prev. Med.* 26: 144-53.

Hanahan, D. and R.A. Weinberg. 2001. The hallmarks of cancer. *Cell* 100: 57-70.

Hartmann, A., H. Blaszyk, J.S. Kovach, and S.S. Sommer. 1997. The molecular epidemiology of P53 gene mutations in human breast cancer. *Trends Genet.*13: 27-33.

Harvard Health Letter. 2003. Hooked on fish? There might be some catches. Health-conscious people eat it three, even four times a week. But farm-raised fish and worries about mercury contamination are churning the waters. 283 (January): 4-5.

Hill, K.A. and S.S. Sommer. 2002. P53 as a mutagen test in breast cancer. *Environmental and Molecular Mutagenesis* 39: 216-227.

Hollstein, M., B. Shomer, M. Greenblatt, T. Soussi, E. Hovig, R. Montesano, and C.C. Harris. 1996. Somatic point mutations in the P53 gene of human tumors and cell lines: Updated compilation. *Nucleic Acids Res.* 24: 141-146.

International Human Genome Sequencing Consortium. 2001. Initial sequencing and analysis of the human genome. *Nature* 409: 860-921.

Key, T.J., P.K. Verkasalo, and E. Banks. 2001. Epidemiology of breast cancer. *The Lancet Oncology* 2: 133-140.

Kitcher, P. 2001. *Science, Truth, and Democracy.* Oxford: Oxford University Press.

Kovach, J.S., A. Hartmann, H. Blaszyk, et al. 1996. Mutation detection by highly sensitive methods indicates that P53 gene mutations in breast cancer can have important prognostic value. *Proc Natl Acad Sci USA* 93: 1093-1096.

Lacey, J.V., Jr., S.S. Devesa, and L.A. Brinton. 2002. Recent trends in breast cancer incidence and mortality. *Environmental and Molecular Mutagenesis* 39, iss. 2-3: 82-88.

Lerner, B.H. 2001. *The Breast Cancer Wars: Hope, Fear, and the Pursuit of a Cure in Twentieth-Century America.* Oxford: Oxford University Press.

Li, J., Z. Zhang, J. Rosenzweig, Y.Y. Wang, and D.W. Chan. 2002. Proteomics and bioinformatics approaches for identification of serum biomarkers to detect breast cancer. *Clin Chem.* 48: 1296-304.

Olsen, O. and P.C. Gøtzsche. 2001. Cochrane review on screening for breast cancer with mammography. *The Lancet* 358: 1340-1342.

Petricoin III, E. F., A.M. Ardekani, B.A. Hitt, P.J. Levine, V.A. Fusaro, S.M. Steinberg, G.B. Mills, C. Simone, D.A. Fishman, E.C. Kohn, and L.A. Liotta. 2002. Use of proteomic patterns in serum to identify ovarian cancer. *The Lancet* 359: 572-577.

Petricoin, E.F.,III, D.K. Ornstein, C.P. Paweletz, A. Ardekani, P.S. Hackett, B.A. Hitt, A. Velassco, C. Trucco, L. Wiegand, K. Wood, C.B. Simone, P.J. Levine, W.M. Linehan, M.R. Emmert-Buck, S.M. Steinberg, E. C. Kohn and L.A. Liotta. 2002. Serum proteomic patterns for detection of prostate cancer. *J Natl Cancer Inst.* 94: 1576-8.

Prehn, A., C. Clarke, B. Topol, S. Glaser, and D. West. 2002. Increase in breast cancer incidence in middle-aged women during the 1990s. *Ann Epidemiol.* 12: 476-81.

Thomas, D.B., D.L. Gao, R.M. Ray, et al. 2002. Randomized trial of breast self-examination in Shanghai: Final results. *J Natl Cancer Inst.* 94: 1445-1457.

van de Vijver, M.J., Y.D. He, L.J. van 't Veer, H. Dai, A.A.M. Hart, D.W. Voskuil, G.J. Schreiber, J.L. Peterse, C. Roberts, M.J. Marton, M. Parrish, D. Atsma, A. Witteveen, A. Glas, L. Delahaye, T. van der Velde, H. Bartelink, S. Rodenhuis, E.T. Rutgers, S.H. Friend, and R. Bernards. 2002. A gene-expression signature as a predictor of survival in breast cancer. *N Engl J Med.* 347: 1999-2009.

van 't Veer, L.J., H. Dai, van de Vijver, M.J. Yudong, D. He, A.A.M. Hart, M. Mao, H.L. Peterse, K. van der Kooy, M.J. Marton, A.T. Witteveen, G.J. Schreiber, R.M. Kerkhoven, C. Roberts, P.S. Linsley, R. Bernards, and S.H. Friend. 2002. Gene expression profiling predicts clinical outcome of breast cancer. *Nature* 415: 530-536.

Venter, J.C., M.D. Adams, E.W. Myers, et al. 2001. The sequence of the human genome. *Science* 291: 1304-1351.

Ziegler, R.G., R.N. Hoover, M.C. Pike, A. Hildesheim, A.M. Nomura, D.W. West, A.H. Wu-Williams, L.N. Kolonel, P.L. Horn-Ross, and J.F. Rosenthal. 2001. Migration patterns and breast cancer risk in Asian-American women. *Journal of the National Cancer Institute* 85: 1819-1827.

CHAPTER TEN

LORETTA M. KOPELMAN

CLINICAL TRIALS FOR BREAST CANCER AND INFORMED CONSENT

How Women Helped Make Research a Cooperative Venture

During the 1970s many women with breast cancer began to insist that clinicians deal less paternalistically with them, inform them of treatment options, and let them use their own values to determine which approaches were best. Their demands for better communication and choice had a well-documented impact on the women's movement, the rejection of patriarchal institutions, the patients' rights movement, and the denunciation of the authoritarian medical culture.[1] In this paper I want to examine how these activists also helped to revolutionize the research culture by insisting that it be a cooperative venture. Their leverage was the power to defeat randomized clinical trials (RCTs) that did not include genuine options or consent. This struck at the heart of research practices since the RCT is generally regarded as the gold standard for evaluating alternative interventions.

Many investigators during this period regarded gaining consent to be a misguided requirement. They argued that the women could not understand what was at stake and claimed that incorporating consent and choice would only ruin the structural integrity of the trials (Zelen 1979, 1241). In the 1970s and 1980s, many clinicians also resisted enrolling their patients in trials. These clinicians did not want to communicate the uncertainties about which therapies were best. They feared that informed consent would destroy trust in the doctor-patient relationship, and maintained they should simply pick the therapy that they believed was best for their patients (Taylor 1984, 1361). For some investigators and clinicians who were saturated in a positivistic philosophy of science, it was hard to admit that values were integral to science and needed to be justified. Consequently, the women's demands for respect of their perspective seemed unreasonable.

This is a philosophical paper about *why it is rational to insist that research be a cooperative venture* and uses this example about women's demand for better

M.C. Rawlinson and S. Lundeen (eds.), The Voice of Breast Cancer in Medicine and Bioethics, 133-161.

communication of options by clinicians about early breast cancer trials and more respect for their right to give consent to illustrate why research needs to be a cooperative venture. A *cooperative venture* requires good communication, including informed consent and respect for the views of the clinicians, investigators, and subjects since each can defeat the studies. If clinicians do not think their patients will get good treatments, they should not agree to enroll their subjects. If women do not trust the clinicians or investigators to communicate the pertinent information and provide good care, they should not consent to participate. If investigators believe that the study is poorly designed or likely to be undermined by biases, they should not agree to do the study.

Good RCTs were badly needed to get the information about how to best treat breast cancer, yet some investigators saw informed consent from potential subjects as an impediment. As informed consent policy took hold, however, several RCT designs were proposed as a means to conduct breast cancer studies. I want to show which schemas are compatible with established moral and legal policy on informed consent and which are not. As women with breast cancer refused to participate, they defeated the trials, helping to make research into a more cooperative venture among investigators, clinicians, and patients. To avoid charges of importing later views into the discussion, I generally use articles from before 1990. After discussing the background to this revolution, the nature of RCTs, and the consent requirements, I will look at some schemas and how they attempted to include informed consent. I will show that some are compatible with these consent requirements and people's desires to be informed partners and some are not. That is, some schemas are not acceptable given the consent requirements or people's desire to be partners in research as a cooperative venture.

BACKGROUND

In the late 1960s most surgeons performed radical mastectomy on their patients with breast cancer, a treatment developed early in the century by Hopkins surgeon William Stewart Halsted. In 1968, 70 percent of the women diagnosed with this disease had this surgery that removed the breast, lymph nodes, and chest wall muscles on the side the cancer was diagnosed. Clinicians believed this gave women their best chance of "cure" (five-year survival), at no real loss, since, in their view, the breast of an older woman was entirely expendable (Lerner 2001, 89, 251). Beginning in the 1970s, these views changed very gradually, with many clinicians still clinging to these beliefs into the 1990s, long after information gained from a series of RCTs showed Halsted's approach as unnecessarily mutilating and disabling. (Clinicians' method of removing large areas of tissue applied to other cancers. Men with prostate cancer had surgeries routinely leaving them incontinent and impotent; these approaches were also found to be unnecessarily mutilating.)

My interest in this topic stemmed from being one of several speakers in May, 1981, for a Medicine Grand Rounds at Brody School of Medicine entitled, "Randomized Clinical Trials: Consent and the Therapeutic Relationship." The section head of hematology-oncology, the late Spencer Raab, M.D., organized the conference; he was an advocate of patients' rights and for newer, less mutilating approaches. I was asked to speak on the "new" informed consent requirements for therapy and research. Many surgeons, investigators, and oncologists expressed impassioned disagreements about whether they could, in good conscience, recommend or perform anything but the Halsted's radical mastectomy. They questioned the rationality of the various treatment options, the need for RCTs, and the possibility of genuine consent from most people. Many of the views I heard that day squared with the results of a survey of doctors published three years later. It documents clinicians' misgivings about entering eligible patients in a nationwide RCT of treatments for breast cancer:[2]

> Physicians who did not enter all eligible patients offered the following explanations: (1) concern that the doctor-patient relationship would be affected by a randomized clinical trial (73 percent); (2) difficulty with informed consent (38 percent); (3) dislike of open discussions involving uncertainty [i.e., telling of random assignments or of the uncertainty about which treatment is best] (22 percent); (4) perceived conflicts between the roles of scientist and clinician (18 percent); (5) practical difficulties in following procedures (9 percent); and (6) feelings of personal responsibility if the treatments were found to be unequal (8 percent). (Taylor 1984, 1363)

Getting clinicians to agree to participate and women to enroll in RCTs was a crucial step toward showing that other treatments were better than Halsted's radical mastectomy. Investigators had to convince skeptical clinicians to enroll their patients in clinical trials when many doctors believed the radical mastectomy was necessary to give their patients the best chance of survival. Many clinicians were so convinced radical mastectomy was best that they resisted even informing women of other options, let alone enrolling them in RCTs. The difficulty was that to get the information needed to change the standard of care for breast cancer, clinicians had to be willing to enter their eligible patients into RCTs. Could they do this in good conscience if they believed, as many did, that radical mastectomy was best for their patients? In their view, they had a duty to provide what *they* believed was the *best* treatment for their patients. This paternalistic attitude annoyed both investigators (how did they know it was best?) and an increasing number of women (don't they have a say about what is best for them?). To enroll patients and get consent, women had to be told that clinicians did not know which of several treatments were best. While some clinicians and patients welcomed and even insisted upon this openness, others found this uncertainty unsettling. Part of what changed was that women became increasingly informed about the controversies swirling in the medical literature about the best treatments at the same time that consent policy took root. Consequently, investigators and clinicians had to make room for good informed consent. During the late 1970s and early 1980s, physician-investigator Bernard Fisher convinced both the physicians to enroll patients and women with breast cancer to enter RCTs (Lerner 2001, 6; Fisher et al. 2002, 567 ff).

Ultimately, Fisher would show that removal of only the tumor or the breast, with or without radiation therapy, resulted in a survival rate comparable to that achieved with Halsted's much more drastic operation. Fisher's findings eventually spelled the end to the radical mastectomy, but also proved a theory long seen as heretical: namely, most breast cancers, by the time they were detected, had already spread throughout the body. Accordingly, chemotherapy, which treats this systemic or metastatic disease, was more important than local surgery or radiation for achieving a cure period (Lerner, 2001, 6; Fisher et al. 2002, 567).

In the case of breast cancer, discrepancies within the mechanistic Halsted model had led Fisher and other researchers to hypothesize and then establish an alternative biological paradigm. Fisher acknowledged how activists within and later outside of the medical profession had pushed physicians to perform better studies and then revise long held assumptions and beliefs. Lerner writes, "Physicians themselves appreciated how the combination of factors—Fisher's data, the growing availability of effective radiotherapy and chemotherapy, and the expectations of women with breast cancer—had induced them to change their ways" (Lerner 2001, 229). With debates raging about what was best in their own literature, many clinicians eventually saw that they were arbitrarily imposing their values about what was "best" on their patients.

The part of the problem I want to consider is how informed consent was woven into RCTs in a way that maintained the RCTs' structural integrity and met the demands of women who wanted information and options. It took their activism, along with information from RCTs, to defeat the prevailing paternalistic and conservative attitudes about the radical mastectomy. After clarifying what RCTs are, the consent policy, and doctors' concerns, I will consider the evolution of RCT designs devised by investigators to accommodate consent and bolster poor accrual rates.

RANDOMIZED CLINICAL TRIALS

Since the 1970s, RCTs have been acknowledged as one of the most important methods for making progress in medical science; some would say it is the most important way to compare the efficacy and safety of different interventions (Fletcher 1979; Gordon 1978; Bonchek 1979; DeVita 1978; Zelen 1979; Angell 1984; Vaisrub 1985). RCTs are prospective controlled studies in which patients are assigned to treatments by a chance mechanism such that when a patient is registered, neither investigators nor patients know which of the treatments will be used. The RCT's research advantage stems from this random assignment because it can eliminate the effects of nuisance variables like age, nutritional habits, or placebo effects in correlating the variable under investigation with observed effects. RCTs do not rely on historical controls (data obtained from chart reviews or literature searches).

Many nonrandomized prospective trials (trials that do not use chance to assign patients to different therapies) rely on historical controls. Historical controls are often viewed as biased or unreliable because data are collected or recorded differently, the natural history of the disease may have changed, the therapy may be given under different circumstances, there may be new or different diagnoses or selection criteria, or placebo effects may be different in different settings. The use of historical controls, then, generally offers less adequate assurances than concurrent controls when the control and test groups are comparable (Vaisrub 1985, 3145). Some non-randomized prospective trials, however, do not use historical controls. These include matching similar subjects into the test and control groups, or blocking comparable groups of subjects into the test and control groups. In addition, non-random assignment in prospective trials may use sequential assignment to maximize the efficiency of the study and achieve statistical significance as soon as possible (Weinstein 1974). A sequential "play-the-winner" rule, for example, may be used when patients enter the trial one-by-one, and when the response is dichotomous (Zelen 1969, 131; Wei 1978, 840).

Non-randomized prospective trials are generally seen as inferior because these comparisons are more likely to have biases affecting how patients react to treatments (Vaisrub 1985; Angell 1984; Kopelman 1983, 1986; for more recent discussions see Kopelman 2004a, 2004b, and Schaffner 2004). This is not to say, of course, that all biases can be entirely eliminated from RCTs. They cannot entirely be eliminated since people's values and preferences are deeply embedded in the choice of which studies to fund, when to begin and end studies, what measures will be used, how groups are established, and so on. Yet RCTs are very good at eliminating or minimizing many biases.

The moral debate about RCTs does not challenge their social utility or scientific merits; rather it questions the extent to which they may compromise other values including patients' rights and welfare or physicians' duties to provide the best treatments available. Critics argue that these rights and duties are more important than making medical progress by means of RCTs. After discussing some of the consent requirements, I will review the debate among critics and defenders of RCTs during the late 1970s and 1980s about the justification for conducting RCTs.

CONSENT

Although there was resistance in practice, a stable moral and legal policy on informed consent for research, therapy, and therapeutics research had emerged in the 1970s (Katz 1972; *Canterbury v. Spence* 1972; Faden et al. 1986). According to this policy, when seeking informed consent for therapy or therapeutic research such as RCTs, clinicians needed to reveal all information they knew, or should have known, that would be regarded as important to those people making the decision. Those seeking consent, for example, should provide patients with information about the diagnosis and prognosis so that the patients understand the disease process. Reasonable alternative treatment options should also be explained, along with their nature, duration, costs, side affects, and potential harms or benefits. The patients should also be told the likely consequences of no treatment.

Even clinicians willing to obtain informed consent, however, were sometimes puzzled about how much information was enough. Two clear legal standards emerged during the 1970s; although since that time, they have gradually come to the same thing in practice. The older standard is the *professional community standard*, which requires that clinicians reveal what qualified medical practitioners in the same field would regard as appropriate to tell patients under similar circumstances. The more recent *reasonable person standard* does not focus on what clinicians are inclined to do, (which was sometimes exceedingly paternalistic), but requires the clinician to reveal any information that a reasonable person would consider material or important to reaching the decision about whether to consent.

The person who gives consent must not only be adequately informed, but must also have the capacity to make decisions. In the recent literature, the terms "competent" and "incompetent" are often reserved for legal terms. The legal presumption is that adults are legally competent and minors are not, however, the courts can rebut this assumption. Most women with breast cancer are legally competent adults with the capacity to make their own health-care decisions.[3]

Consent must also be voluntary or freely given and not manipulated or coerced. The fact that the patients may be distraught does not make them unable to give consent. In health care decision-making several capacities seem especially important for making such health-care decisions. The individuals should not only be able to understand information needed to make informed consent, but also to evaluate this information in terms of stable personal values. In addition, one should be able to use and manipulate the information in a reasonable or at least not irrational way (President's Commission 1982; Kopelman 1990, 2004a, 2004b; Gert et al. 1997).[4]

Clinicians should assess how well the people responsible for giving their consent can deliberate, make and defend choices, understand and use the salient information, and communicate their choices. These features should help clinicians decide if people have the necessary decision-making capacity for important health care decisions. Many authors writing about how to understand decision-making capacity came to favor a sliding scale[4] such that the lower the probability and magnitude of the risk, the less the clinician need scrutinize the decision-making capacity of the person giving consent. But the greater the probability and risk of harm from the person's decision, the higher the duty of clinicians to determine if the person's decision is irrational. If the patient is not competent or lacks the capacity to make decisions, clinicians may have a legal and moral duty to seek a court order so that the courts can authorize the needed intervention.

People's informed consent, then, should have the following elements (See President's Commission for the Study of Ethical Problems and Biomedical and Behavioral Research 1982, 1983; Beauchamp et al. 1991; Faden et al. 1986):

1. People receive all information material or important to their decision.
2. They comprehend or understand the information that has been disclosed.
3. They agree voluntarily to participate.
4. They are competent to make a decision to participate.
5. They agree to the procedure, act, intervention, or research.

In some cases informed consent may be waived, as for incompetent persons, or in personal or public health emergencies.

Not surprisingly, consent for research has additional requirements including a description of the study's nature, purpose, duration, procedures, foreseeable risks, and benefits. In addition, clinicians and investigators must discuss alternative procedures, confidentiality protection, the institution's policy regarding compensation, whom to contact if there are questions or injuries, the voluntary nature of participation, and the right to withdraw from the study. For Institutional Review Boards (IRBs) to ensure that guidelines are followed, statements about risks related to pregnancy or other pertinent patient conditions, such as additional costs and special circumstances for withdrawing from the study (e.g., the danger of abrupt withdrawal from certain drugs) may be required. When these requirements would be inappropriately exacting, the federal regulations allow IRBs to modify or even waive the investigator's obligation to gain consent or obtain a signed consent form (U.S. 1981, 46.117c; 45CFR 46). To do this, the IRB must judge that reasonable persons would have no objection to gathering the information sought, that laws concerning invasion of privacy would not be violated, and that the procedure does not normally require consent. Institutions may lose their federal funding or face legal action if they do not apply these guidelines rigorously.

IRBs became more active and effective in the 1970s due to a series of scandals and increasingly more rigorous guidelines (see Levine 1980, 1986). Although consent policy for research, as well as therapy, solidified in the 1970s, there was considerable skepticism about how meaningful it was to try to seek informed consent from patients for therapy, research or therapeutic research. It was very common to hear such comments as, "People do not want to understand, they just want to feel better." Investigators and clinicians also commented that it was "a waste of time," that "patients cannot really understand," or that "it is meaningless, I can get them to consent to anything." These global assumptions were incorrect and people did want to understand their options, give consent, and have their own values control choices about their lives (Lerner 2001, 14). RCTs are an extremely powerful way to eliminate bias and prejudice, but they are by no means so ideal that the civil rights to consent or to refuse to be used as an object of study should be set aside. One's role as a person is acknowledged through consent.

DOES A DILEMMA EXIST?

In the late 1970s and early 1980s both critics and defenders of RCTs argued that a choice had to be made between conducting good RCTs and honoring patients' rights to consent or doctors' duties. Some RCT proponents argued that these alleged patients' "rights" or doctors' "duties" were unrealistic and/or less important then conducting RCTs and making rapid medical advances (Zelen 1979). In contrast, critics of RCTs held that these rights or duties were genuine and more important than medical advances through research. In their view some potentially important RCTs should not be conducted (Wickler 1981).

I questioned the shared assumption that these critics and defenders of RCTs held, namely that RCTs are incompatible with socially sanctioned patients' rights and doctors' duties (Kopelman 1983, 1986). Some RCTs were morally problematic, but some were not and were compatible with honoring patients' rights and doctors' duties. This presupposes both that doctor's duties are not simply a matter of choosing what they happen to think is best, and that informed consent can be obtained without necessarily undercutting the structural integrity of RCTs. Those who maintained that a dilemma existed questioned both these assumptions. Consequently, to avoid the so-called dilemma we must show *first* that doctors' duties do not preclude recommending RCTs to patients, and *second,* that good consent can sometimes be worked into RCTs without undermining their structural integrity.

THE THERAPEUTIC OBLIGATION

Some doctors believed that they had a therapeutic obligation that was incompatible with enrolling their patients in RCTs. These doctors believed *they* had a duty to select the *best* treatment for *each* patient. Physicians do not usually decide between what seems to them to be equally good therapies by a chance method; rather, they find grounds for preferring one, perhaps because of their own skills or because of the patient's situation or preferences. Other doctors objected to being less than entirely candid with patients about what they regarded to be best for them. The therapeutic relationship is a fiduciary one, so patients have a legitimate interest in their physician's convictions about what treatment is in their best interest. Critics of RCTs argued that if physicians participate in an RCT, they might be less candid about stating these beliefs or deviating from the research protocol, so assigning treatments by a chance mechanism defeats individualized care. They raised troubling charges that to get the best data, good patient care is sometimes compromised by enthusiasm for doing RCTs, and for continuing them until the probability is less than 0.05 that the results could have occurred by chance (Fried 1974; Levine 1980, 1986).

Over time, many clinicians saw that their hunches about what was best were sometimes completely wrong, both in the sense RCTs proved them wrong and in that patients wanted to have options. Many clinicians, as noted, refused to participate in a long-term, multi-institutional RCT that sought to compare mastectomy to limited surgery and radiotherapy as treatments for early breast cancer (Taylor 1984). They were convinced that radical mastectomy always offered better tumor control and survival outcome, well worth the poor cosmetic results. Many even refused to tell women under their care of the choices because of their strong conviction that the "lumpectomy" was inadequate treatment. In Massachusetts the public responded by passing a law *requiring* that surgeons tell women of these alternative treatments and other states passed similar legislation (Lerner 2001, 233). Studies showed, of course, that these surgeons' sincere convictions were wrong (Harris 1985, 1365; Fisher 1985, 665; Lerner 2001, 251).

Informed consent policy quite reasonably requires that physicians must not simply be guided by what they sincerely happen to believe is the best treatment, but must inform patients of recognized risks, benefits, and alternative therapies (Miller 1980; *Canterbury v. Spence* 1972). Whether or not an RCT is contemplated, then, physicians must distinguish their hunches or personal beliefs from more stable evidence and prevailing professional judgments. This ought to give them a basis for saying whether or not therapies are comparable. It would be unreasonable of clinicians to put their own hunches or personal beliefs ahead of reliable data in making decisions about what information and recommendations to pass on to patients (Kopelman 1983, 1ff). Later, Freedman (1987, 141) made the same point in arguing that a moral requirement for conducting RCTs should be that investigators and clinicians can truthfully assure potential subjects that arms of the study are in clinical equipoise, or that there is no known advantage or disadvantage to any group assignment at the start of the trial.

Some clinicians, moreover, insisted it was bad for patients to discuss any uncertainties regarding treatment options with their doctors. These clinicians held that this might compromise a physician's effectiveness either by weakening the patient's trust, hope and morale, or by diminishing doctors' authority or charisma (Taylor 1984, 1363). Even at the time, such reasoning seemed suspect in light of the hot debates about what treatments were most effective (Fisher 1980; NSABP 1985; Lerner 2001, 91; Kopelman 1983, 1ff; 1986, 317ff). In order to fulfill consent requirements even for therapy alone, however, patients needed to be told about whatever uncertainties existed that a reasonable person would consider important in making decisions (Canterbury v. Spence 1972; Faden et al. 1986). Those who recommend a treatment as the best when they do not know this are not being truthful and leave themselves open to the charge that they are not candid enough to admit to their patients they do not know which treatment is best.

During this period, Jay Katz (1984) argues that physicians deny uncertainty as a defense against having to deal with uncertainty with patients. He claims that it is denial because their conscious reasons do not fulfill the goals they propose. He argues that in the long run, the short term benefit of gaining trust or hope by a lack of candor defeats real trust and hope. Communication, Katz argues, is the best way to build genuine trust and hope. He also considers the argument that it costs too much in time to have frank discussions, but finds it unconvincing. These discussions are, he holds, an essential feature of medical practice. They should not be sacrificed, especially considering the high percentage of unnecessary procedures for which our society is willing to pay.

Another concern expressed by doctors for refusing to participate in RCTs is that they might be uncomfortable if their patients are assigned to an arm that turns out to be less successful in combating their disease than others. It would be a mistake to dismiss this worry completely as unjustified paternalism on the grounds that the subjects gave consent. There is a legitimate concern that RCTs might be planned to continue too long. Reasonable people may also disagree about when studies should be stopped early, given early trends. If studies are stopped too quickly, then errors are more likely to result, setting false standards of care; if they are continued too long, then some subject-patients may be harmed or denied optimal care.

Investigators, review boards, physicians, and patients may sincerely disagree whether the arms are in clinical equipoise or whether sufficient reasons exist to stop a study. For one thing, their interests may be radically different. Investigators concerned with discrete outcome measures, such as survival in cancer treatments, may regard two therapies as equivalent when their side effects are very different. Patients are likely to have a greater interest in how therapies affect them personally, such as how sick they will feel (McNeil 1978). Physicians sometimes avoid RCTs because they do not wish to get in the middle (Taylor 1984). Moreover, investigators, panels and journal editors typically require a probability of at least 0.05 as a ground for holding "sufficient reason" exists to believe the groups in the different arms of the study are different. But the 0.05 probability standard, although a reasonable and well-established convention, is nonetheless a moral choice. Wickler writes, "its appropriateness derives from the (moral) evaluation of the human consequences of adopting it" (Wikler 1981, 438). Patients balancing values differently might want to know information regarded as "inconclusive" or as an "early trend" by those investigators who simply define "sufficient reason" as the 0.05 probability standard (Kopelman 1983, 1986).

Continuing a study until the probability of error is less than a probability of 0.05 is considered important and affects how studies are perceived by colleagues, editors, and funding agencies (Vaisrub 1985). One advantage of carefully-watched large studies is that data is obtained quickly and the studies are stopped if a clear disadvantage to one of the arms is shown. Still, though prepared to end studies early if they compromise patient care, some investigators and panelists tenaciously view any differences between treatment arms which have not yet reached statistical significance at the level of 0.05 probability as an early trend or incomplete data base. Yet the threshold of significance of a 0.05 probability is a convention with moral implications (Wickler 1981; Kopelman 1983). Many of our momentous life choices are made on less exacting standards, so the reasonable person might want to learn of early trends. Failure to end studies early, when it is appropriate, risks eroding the kind of trust necessary to make subjects and clinicians willing to participate (Fried 1974).

To support RCTs, clinicians had to come to terms with the problem of when and how studies should be ended. In light of consent policy, some wanted to know at what point preliminary trends would keep a reasonable person from participating (Veatch 1982). According to the federal guidelines (from this period and later) it may be appropriate to inform subjects of "...significant new findings developed during the course of the research which may relate to the subject's willingness to continue participation...." (U.S. 1981, 46.116[b]5; see also the more recent 45 CFR 46).[5]

On a related point, some doctors objected to enrolling their patients in RCTs on the grounds that to do so would create a tension between a doctor's role as clinician and as a scientist or investigator (Taylor 1984). If the patient was not doing well on one arm, the doctor *as clinician* might want to switch the patient, but the doctor *as scientist* might not want to disrupt the study. Critics argued that treatment choices for patients should be swift and individualized, based on what is in the patient's best interest alone, given available treatment, without thought of what a research protocol dictates. This tension between the doctors' role as clinician and investigator remains an important concern, of course, as does the problem of when to end studies if early trends show clear advantages or disadvantages. Despite general agreement that advances in medical knowledge cannot come at the expense of good patient care or the right of informed persons to refuse participation in research, there was sustained disagreement about how to implement these policies. I argued that if a reasonable person would be interested in early trends, or results, or how studies will be ended, then policies should be discussed openly when subject consent is sought (Kopelman 1986, 317ff). Doctors should justify that they are fulfilling fiduciary their duties to patients, including being able to truthfully state that therapies in the different arms of the study are equally acceptable as the trial begins. In some cases patients find the different therapies in the arms of the studies to be in equipoise and are indifferent about their assignment; in other cases patients may identify enough with the purposes of the study that, out of altruism, they accept the assigned therapy whether or not they have some non-medical preference for another (Veatch 1982). Patients need to be assured, however, that their interests are put ahead of the research.

Critics such as Zelen (1979) questioned if such difficult matters regarding treatment options and when to halt trials could ever be reasonably discussed with prospective subjects. These critics did not see that patients, clinicians, and investigators were capable of working together as partners with candor, respect, and trust about the means and goals of the enterprise. Some agreed it was possible, but questioned if enough people could have these discussions to make it possible to conduct sound clinical trials.

Events have shown that many patients were willing to take some risks and suffer some inconveniences. Cancer patients on RCT protocols that I have talked to seem to stoically accept the uncertainties of treatment, taking comfort in the confidence they have in their oncologist to look out for their best interest. They express their debt to earlier generations who helped them, and want to help future patients. In addition, even if there is an additional burden to patients from learning about uncertainty and choice, the burden could be offset by the benefit that can come from believing that they may help the next generation of patients as the last generation helped them.

Women with breast cancer increasingly objected to the lack of good communication about their options and choices. They wanted the opportunity to consent or refuse participation in RCTs, and consequently, some way had to be found to incorporate consent. RCTs create special problems about how or when to inform, or what information to make available during or after trials. But as we shall see in the next section, some RCTs are intrinsically morally troubling from the standpoint of gaining informed consent, and women who were asked to participate in breast cancer trials were reluctant to enroll in those that were problematic.

ALTERNATIVE SCHEMAS

In the later 1970s and early 1980s both many critics of and advocates for RCTs shared a common assumption that I will challenge. They believed that seeking rigorous consent from patients was likely to undermine the structural integrity of RCTs. Some advocates for RCTs, such as Zelen (1979) maintained that informed consent was not needed because it was sufficient that women received good care for their disease. On his view, regulations that they must be told about the nature and purpose of the study were unnecessary. One might state their objection as follows: If rigorous consent is sought for RCTs then the likelihood increases that biases will be introduced as (1) distinct groups favor particular treatments, (2) accrual rate will be slow, or (3) some may drop-out. Any of these circumstances could affect the reliability of the RCT or create problems for the analysis of the data. But if one of these circumstances undermines the integrity of RCTs then arguably it is better not to conduct them." These advocates reached the conclusion that it is better to make medical progress than to stand by some rigorous informed consent standard that defeats RCTs (Zelen 1979). Others, as noted, believed the RCTs were expendable because they conflicted with more important considerations relating to patients' rights or doctors' duties (Wickler 1981).

To answer both sets of critics, I will consider several designs for RCTs seeking to give due consideration to gaining consent for research while maintaining the structural integrity of RCTs.[6] I begin with several schemas where defenders claim that some or all elements of informed consent from potential subjects for RCTs participation may be waived.

(1) RCTs Seeking No Consent

This schema enrolls patients without their consent (see figure 1). A reasonable person would generally not mind waiving consent when treatments do not require it, or where it would be burdensome to obtain, and the research involves very small physical or psychosocial risks of harm.[7] Some early RCTs for breast cancer did not obtain consent (Fried 1974). Advocates for such RCTs argued that patients should be guaranteed good treatments but objected to gaining consent for an RCT. Investigators and clinicians, they argued, were far better able than patients to evaluate alternative treatments in a prospective study, including judging if there was any advantage to being enrolled in one of the arms of the study when compared to others. Studies that did not obtain consent from patients who were subjects in studies became the focus of criticism (Fried 1974). First, objections arose on a rising tide of commitment to informed consent policy. Obtaining consent respects people's rights to make choices for themselves and to control what happens to their bodies. It also gives each subject a role as a person in the study when reasonable people would want to consider whether to be in the study; otherwise they are treated simply as objects of a study. In addition, to allow studies with hazards and life-altering effects to be conducted without obtaining patients' consent would undercut a web of civil liberties that honor people's rights of self-determination and recognize the social utility of such liberties. Consequently, if this policy that does not seek consent were generally adopted and endorsed, it could seriously erode other civil rights. Another practical matter is that some subjects are likely to find out and become angry with the investigators and institutions sponsoring the research. Indeed, during this period there were some lawsuits. In addition, not everyone agrees about what breast cancer therapies are equally suitable or when studies should be ended, as noted above, so the reasonable person being considered as a suitable subject would want to give consent.

Despite investigators' warnings that introducing consent would wreak havoc on the integrity of RCTs, important, moral, legal and policy initiatives insisted that it was generally necessary. The federal regulations (U.S., 45 C.F.R. 46) sometimes allow consent requirements to be waived but *not* if (1) a reasonable person would want to consent or decline; (2) there is violation of laws such as those governing confidentiality or privacy; (3) written consent is normally required; (4) the study has treatment alternatives that a reasonable person would want to know about; or (5) there is more than minimal risk to the subject. Though it almost always seems proper to seek consent of some sort, in rare cases investigators might legitimately gain IRB approval to waive consent for RCTs, although generally not in cancer studies. Reasonable persons, however, would want to know about various options for breast cancer and whether they were enrolled in a clinical trial.

Thus this schema, while appropriate for some studies, is inappropriate for studies when most people would want to have a choice and some information about the study. There are occasions when the reasonable person would not mind waiving consent so this schema is not inherently flawed. Yet it is unsuitable for breast cancer studies where many people do want information about options and choices. Investigators have proposed three other schemas (figures 2-4) that avoid consent altogether or that avoid consent about the nature of the study's various arms.

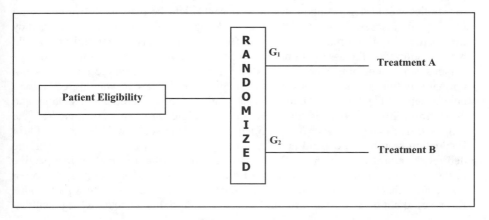

Figure 1:   Randomized research design without consent sought.

(2) Debriefing or Deferred "Consent"

Another schema that does not seek informed consent informs subjects of the study, its nature, and its purpose, only after they have already been enrolled in the study (see figure 2). This schema may usefully be regarded as a variation of the first schema, since if it is ever appropriate to enroll subjects without their consent, it must sometimes be justifiable to tell them afterwards.[8] Randomness of assignment is not distorted by patient choice in the original assignments, since the patients are not asked. Patients or their families are only left the choice of whether to withdraw if the study is ongoing, or to protest based upon the information they are later given.

This design is particularly useful in assessing interventions where consent from the patient or others is not possible. Suppose Emergency Department (ED) or Intensive Care Unit (ICU) personnel need to evaluate emergency procedures, but cannot use historical controls or data from non-emergency care. In some cases an RCT might be the best design, but due to the need to give care quickly, obtaining consent before therapy would compromise patient care. In emergencies there may be no opportunity to seek unpressured consent, yet testing the efficacy of emergency therapies is important (Wolfe and Bone 1977). Unless the testing is controlled, however, it is difficult to obtain reliable and generalizable information since outcomes are affected by differing therapists, techniques, and circumstances. Fost and Robertson proposed merely informing subjects or proxies of the study and deferring gaining consent for no more than 48 hours; they urged rigorous IRB surveillance to protect patients from harm (Fost and Robertson 1980).

Deferred "consent" is not really consent, of course, but more like debriefing. If things go badly, this debriefing might not enhance doctor-patient relations that are often not long standing in EDs and ICUs (Beauchamp 1980). This method is controversial because "consent" is deferred not because of the random method of the assignment. Deferred consent would be no less controversial if a non-random method were used to assign subjects. The evaluation of the suitability of this schema for studies would depend upon whether consent might be reasonably waived using the grounds discussed earlier with figure 1 designs. If all are *standard* emergency treatments, one might make such a case. But to justify waiving consent one would have to show that the assumptions made earlier have been met, e.g. that reasonable persons would not object or that it is the kind of treatment where consent is not normally required. Special consideration is given in the law to waiving consent in emergencies if the person is "unconscious or otherwise incapable of consenting, and harm from failure to treat is imminent and outweighs any harm threatened by the proposed treatments" (*Canterbury v. Spence* 1972, 191; see also Faden et al. 1986). Evaluation would also depend upon the quality of the information given during the debriefing, and if it is given to all who have a claim to the information irrespective of the outcome. To monitor the quality of the information, IRBs might, as they often do, require that a form be signed with a copy going to the consenting party. This form would not be a consent form in the ordinary sense, but an acknowledgment that the patients were informed. Of course, deferred "consent" cannot be justified merely on the grounds that the study could not otherwise be done.

This schema, while justifiable in some situations, would be unsuitable for breast cancer studies where there is time and opportunity to gain consent, and where the reasonable person would want to have these opportunities. The remaining designs seek consent, and I will assume that investigators must do so in accordance with legal and federal guidelines and the moral purposes expressed therein.

(3) Blind and Double Blind Studies

One of the most widely used RCT schemas is represented by figure 3, namely RCT studies that are blind (patients do not know what therapy they get) or the double-blind (neither do those providing therapy).[5] To meet consent requirements, people must understand the nature and purpose of the study, including the fact that if they participate they will not know their therapy or group assignment. So after patient eligibility is determined, the entire protocol should be explained, with patients having the opportunity to consider the risks and benefits of all the treatment arms; patients are then asked to consent without knowledge of their group assignment. If patients agree to participate, then they get randomly assigned to treatments. This design seems most appropriate when, in order to evaluate the therapy, the subjects and/or the clinician-investigators should not know the group assignments even when the study is underway. Drug studies comparing a standard or new drug to another standard drug, to a placebo, or to both, frequently use this schema.

In terms of the consent requirements this design is not problematic if patients or their representatives give consent that is appropriately competent, voluntary, and informed (e.g., that one group will receive a placebo). While non-therapeutic studies can use this design, we are considering *therapeutic* trials, so the requirements made at the beginning of the paper must be met. For example, any placebo used must also meet the null hypothesis and the arms of the study must be in clinical equipoise. Studies of this design (figure 3) will have difficulty attracting sufficient numbers of people if it is important to people to know the treatment modality before they consent. If the refusal rate is high, or if it is reasonable to suppose it would be high, this might lead us to question either whether seeking consent without knowledge of the group assignment is appropriate, or whether there is clinical equipoise of a balance of risks and possible benefits in the different arms of the study.

A statistical difficulty is that this design may lead to skewed patient accrual if distinctive groups of persons decline in greater numbers. The higher the refusal rate, moreover, the more doubtful it becomes that the results of the trial, while internally valid in that all entering subjects were randomized, can be generalized to the entire population of patients. This important and frequently-used design, then, seems appropriate for some studies, but not for others.

Certain breast cancer studies using this schema did not separate the initial screening for cancer from the decision to perform a lumpectomy or mastectomy. Women went into surgery not knowing whether they had cancer or, if they had it,

148   LORETTA M. KOPELMAN

which treatment they would receive.[9] Because of this uncertainty many physicians were reluctant to ask their patients to participate in these studies; and those physicians who agreed found many women unwilling to accept such conditions (Fisher, NSABP, B-06 1980; Taylor 1984; Ellenberg 1984). These trials were a big improvement over similar studies done by other investigators who sought no consent (Fried 1974). But because they sought consent in these trials they had a slow accrual rate and ran the risk of skewed patient accrual affecting general applicability of the results. In response to these problems, some investigators switched to the prerandomized schema represented in figures 4 and 5 (Ellenberg 1984).

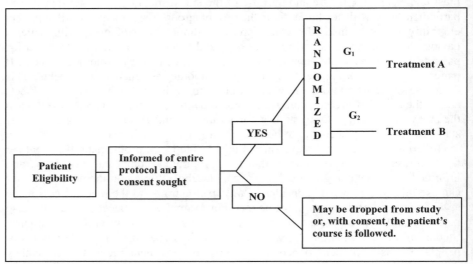

Figure 2:   Randomized research design with consent sought from subjects who are not informed of their group assignment.

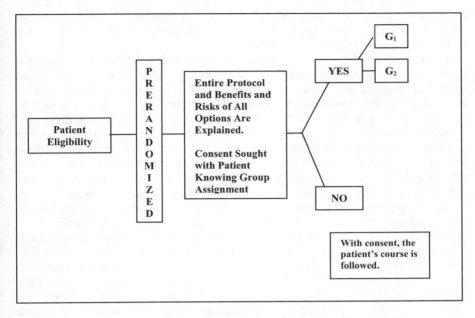

Figure 3:   **Prerandomized design similar to that employed in NSABP B-06 (Fisher). Patient learns of entire protocol, treatment options, and group.**

(4-5) RCTs Using Prerandomization, Informing Some but Not All of Their Group Assignments, Treatment Options, and of the Nature and Purpose of the Study

Zelen proposed the designs depicted in figures 4 and 5, comparing them to figures 1 and 3 (Zelen 1979). In figure 4, after patient eligibility is determined, patients are randomly assigned to groups. Those assigned to one group, G1, receive standard medical care, treatment A, but no consent for the research is sought. Those in the other group, G2, have the entire protocol explained, learning that this is a research project, that patients have been randomly assigned to groups, and that their group can receive the experimental treatment B, while the other group will receive the standard care A. At that time they are asked whether they would be willing to participate in the study and receive the experimental treatment B. They are told they may decline the experimental treatment B and consent for and receive standard treatment A. All those assigned to G2, whether they accept the experimental treatment B or decline it and opt for standard treatment A, know they are part of a study. In contrast, those assigned to G1 do not know they are part of a research study.

One problem with Zelen's design is that the groups are seriously different in at least one way: all patients in G2 know something those in G1 do not, namely, they know about the study. This could affect their responses. Such knowledge might, for example, result in group differences in the compliance rate, or in the therapy's placebo effect, and thus make the two groups, although initially randomized, no longer comparable. Accordingly, how can it be presumed that those getting treatments A and B are "similar" patients?

The second of Zelen's designs, depicted in figure 5, differs from figure 4 designs in that those randomly assigned to G2 are asked to choose whether they would prefer receiving standard treatment A or experimental treatment B. Those selected for G2 might feel less pressured to consent to or decline experimental treatment B, since they do not have to say "no" to the experimental therapy in order to get standard treatment A as those in figure 4 designs; they have merely to choose one or the other therapy. Arguably, studies represented by figure 5 seem preferable to those depicted in figure 4 since they offer patients in the experimental group a less pressured choice between therapies. However, figure 5 schemas may be more problematic to interpret since unique groups may seek particular therapies.

Designs represented by figure 4 and figure 5, however, are morally problematic because subjects in G1 do not know that they are enrolled in a research study. Zelen argues that this is acceptable because patients get standard care. Curran defends Zelen's design, arguing that federal research guidelines allow this because they permit investigators with IRB approval to obtain data without consent from chart reviews (Curran 1979). Fost (1979), Levine (1981), and I (1983, 1986) however, argue that not informing those in G1 fails to serve the moral purpose behind the guidelines and laws supporting people's right to consent. The regulations require telling people the purpose of the study. Moreover, reasonable people might want to know that they are enrolled in a study and of the other therapies. It does not seem that gathering data from Zelen's control groups is like gathering data from chart reviews, because the study is not a thing of the past, and because it affects how their present care is selected. This method, with its lack of candor, also has the potential of eroding trust and weakening a good doctor-patient relationship.

Thus, in terms of the consent requirements, Zelen's designs, figures 4 and 5, seem indefensible unless, like figure 1 designs, it is justifiable to waive consent for those in G1 anyway. If this cannot be done, and it does not seem likely in breast cancer studies, then these designs are inherently flawed. Those in G1 do not give consent and do not know that a study is in progress, and this is problematic because it should and could be obtained. In the next section, designs represented by figure 6 are examined and also found to be unacceptable RCT schemas when judged in relationship to consent requirements.

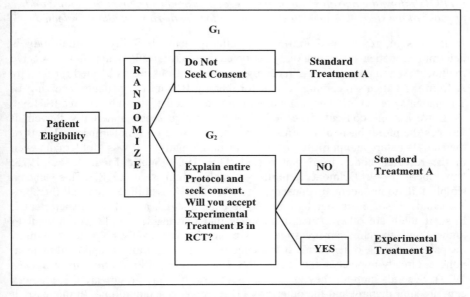

Figure 4: Designed by Zelen (1979) consent for RCT sought only from patients randomly assigned to G_2. After both options are explained, the patient is asked if an experimental treatment is acceptable.

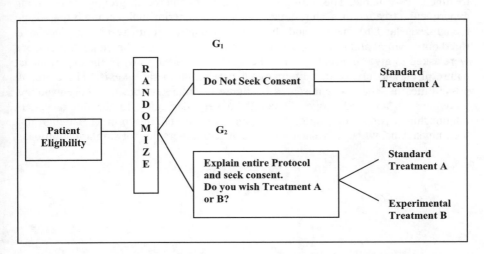

Figure 5: Designed by Zelen (1979) consent for RCT sought only from patients randomly assigned to G_2. They are given the opportunity to choose Treatment A or B after the options are explained.

(6) RCTs informing no subject of multiple group assignments, or of the nature and purpose of the study, but seeking only consent for the therapy randomly selected

In the design, represented in figure 6, after patient eligibility for the study is determined, patients are randomly assigned into groups. Patients in G1 receive treatment A, and patients in G2 receive treatment B. Consent is obtained for therapy A from the patients receiving A, and for therapy B from the patients receiving B. The patients are not told about any other group or that they are subjects in a RCT.

If we assume consent is needed, then this design seems inherently flawed. It violates the moral basis of informed consent because it does not inform subjects of the study's nature and purpose, or of treatment alternatives. It was problematic even in the research codes from that period (U.S. 1981; World Med. Assoc. 1975; Nuremberg 1949; Belmont Report, National Commission 1978). This schema simply fails to get adequate consent. There are three possibilities here: all therapies are standard, some are standard and some experimental, and all are experimental. First, if there are other standard therapies that reasonable people would want to know about, the clinician-investigators are morally and legally obligated to inform the patient of these other standard therapies, and this obligation is supported by legal policies already in place in the 1970s (U.S. 1981; Miller 1980; *Canterbury v. Spence* 1972). Second, suppose they are not all standard, but one group, say G2, receives experimental therapy and the other, say G1, receives a standard one. In this case, it would be a clear violation of the consent policy and its moral grounding if investigators fail to inform them of the study and tell patients in G2 that a standard treatment is available. The third possibility is that some or all groups are receiving experimental treatments. (All groups might get an experimental therapy if there is no recognized standard therapy and the use of a control group receiving placebo is ruled out.) Moral and legal consent requirements would again be violated if persons were asked to give "consent" without being told about the study or the experimental nature of the therapy, or that alternative experimental therapies exist. Therefore, all possibilities in schemas represented by figure 6 violate established consent policy, guidelines or laws. Moreover, it could be very damaging to the doctor-patient relationship if people inadvertently discover (e.g., by talking to other patients) that their physicians, without explanation, give different therapies for similar conditions.

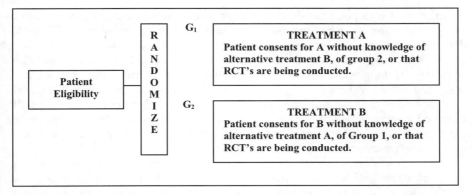

Figure 6: **Randomized research design with consent sought only for specific treatment modality. Subjects are not informed of other groups, alternative treatments, or that an RCT is in progress.**

(7) Prerandomization; RCTs informing all subjects of their group assignment, treatment options, and the nature and purpose of the study, when consent is sought

This schema, represented in figure 7, was used in several nationwide cancer studies to try to solve the problem of slow patient accrual using other designs. Bernard Fisher used it in the study of alternative surgical treatments for Stage 1 breast cancer (NSABP B-06). The project compared total mastectomy to segmental mastectomy, with and without radiation. The design was intended both to answer objections to cancer study designs (like that of figure 2) that did not separate consent for screening and surgery, and to determine which standard therapy was better in terms of long-term survival. It was supposed that if it could be shown, as it was, that they offer comparable outcomes of tumor control with no difference in the survival rate for certain types of breast cancer, then the less disfiguring and invasive procedures would naturally be preferable (Fisher 1985; Harris 1985). The therapies offered in this RCT were standard so that even if the patient declined to participate but sought treatment, she would probably receive one of the treatment options. Thus the investigators were interested in obtaining consent to follow the course of those who refused to participate in the study. Using this design, patient eligibility was determined and, immediately before the informational session, the clinician telephoned the national randomization office for the patient's random assignment to a treatment group. The patient was informed that if she agreed to participate she would receive the treatment that had been randomly selected for her and what that treatment would be. After being so informed, the patient either consented to be part of the study or declined. If the patient did not want to receive the therapy to which she was assigned, she refused at this time and received the treatment of her choice. In that event, she was asked if investigators could follow the results of the treatment she selected.

In contrast with blind and double-blind studies (figure 3), consent is sought with the patient knowing what treatment she will receive, so it is not difficult to determine whether or not persons reject some arm of the study at a greater rate than others since they know their assignment before consent is sought. Another advantage of the prerandomized schema is that all are informed that they are in a study and that other therapies are being tested. Since the entire protocol is explained, they are told of the risks and likely benefits of alternative therapies and are candidly informed that physicians do not know which treatment is preferable. Furthermore, if the prerandomized assignment is unacceptable to the patient, the patient can decline or seek another treatment.

Although it is not inherently flawed, like schemas represented in figures 4 and 5, there are some problems with the schema represented in figure 7 that make it suitable for only some studies. One possible limitation of this schema is that informing bias on the part of clinician-investigators could arise since they know the group assignment before consent is sought. They could have a research interest in convincing the patient of the importance of the RCT and in gaining consent, or might simply be more comfortable concentrating on the likely benefits of the group to which the subject has been assigned. The Fisher study seemed to offset the possible pitfall of bias in informing subjects by providing the same excellent three-page consent form for persons in all groups, clearly setting out the risks and benefits of the alternative treatment modalities. Many women who were reluctant to participate in blind or double blind breast cancer studies agreed to participate in Fisher's study using this design.

A second limitation of this design is that while it worked for Fisher, and there is evidence that physicians and subjects like to use this schema, others have found it very difficult to use. Ellenberg concluded "prerandomization should be considered a last-resort measure...[and] should be abandoned if it does not result in an increase in accrual that is more than sufficient to offset the loss of efficiency inherent in the use of this design" (Ellenberg 1984, 1408). Figure 7 has the potential for creating headaches for statisticians and investigators when there are a lot of refusals. But perhaps a clear pattern of refusals or preferences should make us wonder if there is a genuine balance in the arms of the study. Prerandomized schemas may be useful for some but cannot be used for all RCTs. They cannot be employed, for example, when evaluating therapies that call for blind or double-blind testing.

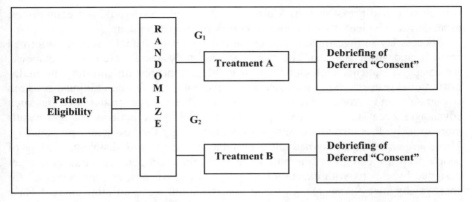

Figure 7:   Debriefing or deferred "consent," proposed to evaluate care when
consent cannot be obtained before trials.

CONCLUDING REMARKS

The purpose of this discussion was to examine the role women with breast cancer have had in encouraging investigators and clinicians to view RCTs as cooperative ventures. In the later 1970s and early 1980s, women defeated studies that they found unacceptable by refusing to enroll. Great progress in treating cancer resulted, in part, from patients' willingness to participate in clinical trials. For research to become a standard of care in oncology, however, some fairly big changes had to occur and some of them were the result of women-activists demanding changes in how patients with breast cancer were treated. For one thing, clinicians had to change their paternalistic approach, set aside their hunches about what was best, admit uncertainties, and share the available options with patients. Women with breast cancer helped to bring these changes about by criticizing the authoritarian medical establishment and demanding genuine options and choices.

Both design and moral problems may arise in planning RCTs, but the criticisms in the 1970s and 1980s that there is an inherent incompatibility between RCT methods and patients' rights, welfare, and a good patient-doctor relationship, does not seem justified. Investigators devised a variety of schemas to fulfill consent requirements. Some tried to avoid or minimize the effects of informed consent because of its potential to distort randomness and introduce nuisance variables. Some of the schemas they proposed (figures 4-6) did not offer information or options a reasonable person would want. As a result, accrual rates were poor. Avoiding some or all of the elements of informed consent that has been worked out in the moral and legal literature, then, was not the answer to getting good enrollment from women. In short, researchers found that RCT schemas ignoring broadly supported patients' rights, such as informed consent, were likely to fail, at least with women who had breast cancer. Moreover, many clinicians would not compromise basic duties to patients by recommending they participate in them.

Success lay in investigators taking the opposite path, namely, seeking informed consent and justifying that the arms of the study were in clinical equipoise. Increasingly, patients and clinicians saw the advantages of enrolling in multi-institutional research using the same protocols, both in offering additional research advantages and added benefits to patients. These large trials have research advantages because they make it possible to enroll more patients and get results more quickly. It is also an advantage to patients to get the best treatments quickly. These large trials also may neutralize bias that can result from distinctive groups of people who use certain institutions. In addition, these cooperative studies often are designed by experts with exacting quality-control provisions, and are reviewed for approval by many agencies; expert panelists should agree to stop them if early results show clear advantages to some assignments. Such large studies can result in improved care for all groups as well as in careful attention to consent requirements. Thus, RCTs can sometimes contribute to careful consent procedures and good patient care as well as the worthiness of studies (Fisher 1985).

In light of important patients' rights and doctors' duties to patients, some RCT designs are inherently flawed, or so I have tried to show. However, both critics and defenders of RCTs who assumed RCT methods were always at odds with consent requirements fail to make their case. Although my interests are philosophical, namely that it is rational to reject certain designs, the reasons given for such rejection seem to mirror what actually happened. In the late 1970s and early 1980s, women demanded that clinicians inform them of options and that clinicians or investigators not simply assign a treatment to them. As we have seen, consent may be incorporated in a variety of ways to accommodate good design and to acknowledge that the patient-subject is a partner in research ventures. The suitability of RCT designs cannot be determined abstractly as they have different strengths and weaknesses in relation both to the consent requirements and the structural integrity of the RCT. Some of the RCT schemas that investigators proposed were not acceptable, given patients' rights and clinicians' duties to patients. So, investigators had to scramble to find acceptable designs that would make studies a more cooperative venture among patients, clinicians, and investigators. Consequently, women with breast cancer have helped transform the way in which clinical trials are conducted and consent is obtained. This is a philosophical paper, but one that relies on a case study about breast cancer research in the late 1970s and early 1980s to underscore the issues about the kind of studies a reasonable person should find acceptable.

Loretta M. Kopelman is Professor and Chair of the Department of Medical Humanities at East Carolina University School of Medicine

NOTES

1. For a comprehensive account and many key references see Barron H. Lerner's, *The Breast Cancer Wars: Hope, Fear, and the Pursuit of a Cure in Twentieth-Century America* (2001). I gratefully acknowledge my use of this research throughout this paper.

2. Many of these concerns have abated in the last two decades as attention to patients' rights, including informed consent, increased. In addition, a variety of research policies and protections bolstered moral arguments that the social utility of research should not be permitted to override patients' rights.

3. For a discussion of research with special or vulnerable groups, such as children and incompetent adults, see Kopelman (2000, 2004a, 2004b).

4. For more recent discussions, see Brock and Buchanan (1989) and Kopelman (1990, 2004a, 2004b).

5. Even where there is no legal requirement to do so, clinician-investigators often feel a moral obligation to inform subjects of early trends, results, or unexpected findings. Until recently, the matter of whether or not to end a study early has relied largely on this good will of the investigators. For some studies, especially those that are risky, it seems reasonable and in accordance with the spirit of the consent requirements that, at the time consent is sought, there be frank discussion of if or when early trends will be reported to subjects, and when or how studies are discontinued. The policy on reporting results could then be included in the informational session and on the consent form. When consent is sought, prospective patient-subjects would learn whether and under what circumstances investigators will inform them of results. This would acknowledge subjects as partners as well as the extent to which participants have some claim to the information before they agree to participate (Kopelman 1983).

6. These figures were discussed in two earlier papers (Kopelman 1983, 1986) but are here applied to the studies of breast cancer. Nonetheless, portions of this paper are similar to these earlier discussions. I have argued and continue to argue that research, including RCTs, should be regarded as a cooperative venture among investigators and subjects (Kopelman 1981, 1983, 1986, 2004a, 2004b).

7. Suppose investigators wish to test which of two routinely used soap solutions offers better protection from post-operative infections. There is no reason to suppose one is better than the other, or that anyone would care which soap was used on them; no results are expected for many months. Should each patient going into surgery at a busy hospital be required to give consent? Some simply assume that any failure to get consent harms or shows disrespect (Ramsey 1970), but this is not obvious (Kopelman 1983, 1986). Here it hardly seems worth the time and effort to gain consent. Such a study might gain IRB approval without consent. Of course what appears to be a very low risk study may not be, and some soaps were found to cause serious harm to premature infants. But this shows why it is important to encourage research and testing of medical practice.

8. Deferred "consent" or debriefing is sometimes used in deception studies that have their own special problems (Mead 1969). For current requirements concerning the use of "deferred" consent see U.S. CFR 45, CFR 46.

9. It was common for this to occur even outside trials. Betty Ford and Happy Rockefeller accepted such an approach (Lerner 2001).

REFERENCES

Almy, T.P. 1977. Therapeutic trials, town and gown, and the public interest. *New England Journal of Medicine* 296: 279-280.

Angell, M. 1984. Patient preferences in randomized clinical trials. *New England Journal of Medicine* 310, no. 21: 1385-1387.

Beauchamp, T.L. 1980. Commentary: The ambiguities of deferred consent. *IRB* 2, no. 7: 6-8.

Beauchamp, T.L., et al. 1991. Ethical guidelines for epidemiologists. *Journal of Clinical Epidemiology*, 44S, no.1: 151S-169S.

Beecher, H.K. 1966. Ethics and clinical research. *New England Journal of Medicine* 274: 1354-1360.

Bonchek, L.I. 1979. Are randomized trials appropriate for evaluating new operations? *New England Journal of Medicine* 301: 44-45.

Buchanan, A.E. and D.W. Brock. 1989. *Deciding for Others: The Ethics of Surrogate Decision Making.* Cambridge, MA: Cambridge University Press.

Canterbury v. Spence. 464 F.2d 722 (D.C. Cir. 1972).

Check, W.A. 1980. Protecting and informing research subjects. *Journal of the American Medical Association* 243: 1985-1993.

Curran, W.J. 1979. Reasonableness and randomization in clinical trials: Fundamental law and governmental regulations. *New England Journal of Medicine* 300: 1273-1275.

DeVita, V.T., Jr. 1978. The evolution of therapeutic research in cancer. *New England Journal of Medicine* 298: 907-910.

Ellenberg, S.S. 1984. Randomized designs in comparative clinical trials. *New England Journal of Medicine* 310: 1404-1408.

Faden, R.R., T.L. Beauchamp, and N.M.P. King. 1986. *History and Theory of Informed Consent.* New York: Oxford University Press.

Fisher, B. 1980. The national surgical adjuvant project for breast and bowel cancer. (NSABP Protocol B-06). Distributed in 1980 to surgeons.

Fisher, B., J.-H. Jeong, S. Anderson, et al. 2002. Twenty-five-year follow-up of a randomized trial comparing radical mastectomy, total mastectomy, and total mastectomy followed by irradiation. *New England Journal of Medicine* 347, no. 8: 567-575.

Fisher, B., M. Bauer, R. Margolese, et al. 1985. Five-year result of a randomized clinical trial comparing total mastectomy and segmental mastectomy with or without radiation in the treatment of breast cancer. *New England Journal of Medicine* 312: 665-673.

Fletcher, R.H. and S.W. Fletcher. 1979. Clinical research in medical journals. *New England Journal of Medicine* 301: 180-183.

Fost, N. 1979. Consent as a barrier to research. *New England Journal of Medicine* 300: 1272-1279.

Fost, N. and J. Robertson. 1980. Deferring consent with incompetent patients in an intensive care unit. *IRB* 2, no. 7: 5-6.

Freedman, B. 1987. Equipoise and the ethics of clinical research. *New England Journal of Medicine* 317, no. 3: 141-145.

Fried, C. 1974. *Medical Experimentation: Personal Integrity and Social Policy*. New York: American Elsevier Publishing Company.

Gert, B., C.M. Culver, and K.D. Clouser. 1997. *Bioethics: A Return to Fundamentals*. New York: Oxford University Press.

Gordon, Jr., R.S. 1978. Clinical trials. *New England Journal of Medicine* 298: 400-401.

Gore, S.M. 1981. Assessing clinical trials--first steps. *British Medical Journal* 282: 1605-1607.

Harris, J.R., S. Hellman, and D.W. Kinne. 1985. Limited surgery and radiotherapy for early breast cancer. *New England Journal of Medicine* 313: 1365-1368.

Hill, A.B. 1963. Medical ethics and controlled trials. *British Medical Journal* 1: 1043-1049.

Jonas, H. 1969. Philosophical reflections on experimenting with human subjects. *Daedalus* 98, no. 2: 219-247.

Katz, J. 1984. Why doctors don't disclose uncertainty. *Hastings Center Report* (February): 35-44.

———— 1972. *Experimentation With Human Beings, Part III*. New York: Russell Sage Foundation.

Kopelman, L.M. 2004a. Research methodology/II. Clinical trials. In *Encyclopedia of Bioethics*, 3rd Edition, ed. Stephen G. Post, 2334-2343. New York: MacMillan Reference USA.

———— 2004b. Research policy/II. Risk and vulnerable groups. In *Encyclopedia of Bioethics*, 3rd Edition, ed. Stephen G. Post, 2365-2372. New York: MacMillan Reference USA.

———— 1990. On the evaluative nature of competency and capacity judgments. *International Journal of Law and Psychiatry* 13, no. 4 (Fall): 309-329.

———— 1986. Consent on randomized clinical trials: Are there moral or design problems? *The Journal of Medicine and Philosophy* 11: 317-345.

———— 1983. Randomized clinical trials, consent and the therapeutic relationship. *Clinical Research* 31, no. 1: 1-11.

———— 1981. Estimating risk in human research. *Clinical Research* 29: 1-8.

Lerner, B.H. 2001. *The Breast Cancer Wars: Hope, Fear, and the Pursuit of a Cure in Twentieth - Century America*. New York: Oxford University Press.

Levine, R.J. 1981. *Ethics and Regulation of Clinical Research*, 1st Edition. Baltimore: Urban and Schwarzenberg Publishing Company.

McCartney, J.J. 1979. A response to Dr. Whitley. *Hastings Center Report* 9, no. 4: 46-47.

———— 1978. Encephalitis and ara-A: An ethical case study. *Hastings Center Report* 8, no. 6: 5-7.

McNeil, B.J., R. Weichselbaum, and S.G. Pauker. 1978. Fallacy of the five year survival in lung cancer. *New England Journal of Medicine* 299: 1397-1401.

Mead, M. 1969. Research with human beings: A model derived from anthropological field research. In *Experimentation with Human Subjects* , ed. P.A. Freund, 152-177. New York: George Braziller Company.

160 LORETTA M. KOPELMAN

Mill, J.S. 1974. *On Liberty.* New York: Penguin Books.

Miller, L.J. 1980. Informed consent I. *Journal of American Medical Association* 244, no. 18: 2100-2103.

Moeschberger, M.L., et al. 1985. Methods of randomization in controlled clinical trials. *American Journal of Emergency Medicine* 3, no. 5: 467-473.

National Commission for the Protection of Human Subjects. 1979. *The Belmont Report, 1979.* Report to the Secretary of the Department of Health, Education, and Welfare. (Now the Department of Health and Human Values). Washington, D.C.

Nuremberg Code. Germany (Territory under Allied Occupation, 1945-1955: U.S. Zone) Military Tribunals. 1947. Permissible medical experiments. In *Trials of War Criminals Before the Nuremberg Tribunals Under Control Law No. 10.* Vol. 2. Washington, D.C.: U.S. Government Printing Office. Available at: http://ohrp.osophs.dhhs.gov/irb/irb_appendices.htm.

President's Commission for the Study of Ethical Problems and Biomedical and Behavioral Research. 1983. *Implementing Human Research Regulations.* Washington, D.C.

President's Commission for the Study of Ethical Problems and Biomedical and Behavioral Research. 1982. *Making Health Care Decisions*, Vol. 1 and Vol. 2. Washington, D.C.

Ramsey, P. 1970. *The Patient as Person.* New Haven, CT: Yale University Press.

Rutstein, D.D. 1969. The ethical design of human experiments. *Daedalus* 98, no. 2: 523-541.

Schaffner, K.F. 2004. Research methodology/I. Conceptual issues. In *Encyclopedia of Bioethics*, 3rd Edition, ed. Stephen G. Post, 2326-2334. New York: MacMillan Reference USA.

Taylor, K.M., R.G. Margolese, and C.L. Soskolne. 1984. Physicians' reasons for not entering eligible patients in a randomized clinical trial of surgery for breast cancer. *New England Journal of Medicine* 310, no. 21: 1363-1367.

Urbach, P. 1982. Randomization and the designs of experimentations. *Philosophy of Science* 52: 256-273.

U.S. Code of Federal Regulations (CFR) 1981. Public welfare final regulations amending basic HHS policy for the protection of subjects. Title 45 CFR 46. *Federal Register* 46, no. 16: 8366-8392.

Vaisrub, N. 1985. Manuscript review from a statistician's viewpoint. *Journal of American Medical Association* 253, no. 21: 3145-3147.

Van Eys, J. 1979. Randomized clinical trials in pediatric oncology. *New England Journal of Medicine* 300: 1115.

Veatch, R. 1982. The patient as partner: Ethics in clinical oncology research. *The Johns Hopkins Medical Journal* 151: 155-161.

Wei, L.J., and S. Durham. 1978. The randomized play-the-winner rule in medical trials. *Journal of the American Statistical Association* 73: 834-840.

Weinstein, M.C. 1974. Allocation of subjects in medical experiments. *New England Journal of Medicine* 291: 1278-1286.

Wexler, N.S., et al. 1985. Huntington's disease homozygotes identified. Abstract. *American Journal of Human Genetics* 37, no. 4 (July Supplement): A82.

Whitley, R.J. 1979. Encephalitis and adenine arabinoside: An indictment without facts. *Hastings Center Report* 9(4), no. 4: 44-46.

Wickler, D. 1981. The ethics of clinical trials. *Seminars in Oncology* 8, no. 4: 437-441.

Wolfe, J.E. and R.C. Bone. 1977. Informed consent in critical care medicine. *Clinical Research* 25: 53-56.

World Medical Association, Declaration of Helsinki. 1964. Recommendations guiding medical doctors and biomedical research involving human subjects. Adopted by the 18th World Medical Assembly, Helsinki, Finland. (Amended in 1975, 1983, 1989, 1996, and 2001).

Zelen, M. 1979. A new design for randomized clinical trials. *New England Journal of Medicine* 300: 1242-1245.

————— 1969. Play the winners role and the controlled clinical trials. *Journal of the American Statistical Association* 64: 131-146.

CHAPTER ELEVEN

ANNE MOYER AND MARCI LOBEL

THE ROLE OF PSYCHOSOCIAL RESEARCH IN UNDERSTANDING AND IMPROVING THE EXPERIENCE OF BREAST CANCER AND BREAST CANCER RISK

Many aspects of breast cancer afford an opportunity for fruitful involvement and investigation by psychosocial researchers and clinicians. Recognition of the psychosocial challenges faced by cancer patients and the emergence of the field of psychosocial oncology have provided roles for social scientists and other behavioral researchers to apply their skills to address important issues. These issues include facilitating treatment decision-making, alleviating treatment side effects, and providing evidence supporting or refuting popular beliefs regarding factors that influence cancer progression, such as an intrepid attitude toward the disease. In this chapter, we highlight important examples of psychosocial research, conducted in the laboratory and in naturalistic settings, that have contributed to an improved understanding of the experience of breast cancer and breast cancer risk. This knowledge empirically informs the development of educational materials, tools to assist in treatment decision-making, and interventions for individuals coping with breast cancer.

DIFFICULTIES ASSOCIATED WITH BEING AT ELEVATED RISK FOR BREAST CANCER

Even women who have not experienced breast cancer may find the prospect of developing the disease extremely worrisome. Although developing breast cancer is a reasonable concern for all women because of its high prevalence, women with a family history of the disease are at elevated risk. There is evidence that women at increased risk, such as those with first-degree relatives with breast cancer, vastly overestimate their risk (Daly et al. 1996). This overestimation is associated with distress, anxiety, and intrusive thoughts about breast cancer on the order of what might be expected in people suffering from post-traumatic stress disorder (Lerman et al. 1994; Thewes et al. 2003). Moreover, distress in these women has been shown to interfere with behaviors critical to early detection of breast cancer, such as

M.C. Rawlinson and S. Lundeen (eds.), The Voice of Breast Cancer in Medicine
and Bioethics, 163-181.

adhering to recommended mammography screening guidelines (Lerman et al. 1993; Schwartz et al. 1999).

Overestimation of risk is fairly intransigent to disconfirming evidence. In a randomized clinical trial involving individualized risk estimates provided by a nurse-educator during counseling sessions, women who were counseled were subsequently more accurate than a control group. However, large proportions of women in both groups still overestimated their risk (Schwartz et al. 2001). In addition, women with high levels of cancer-related distress appeared to be least likely to benefit from the counseling.

A recent laboratory study sheds light on the mechanisms responsible for the difficulty of women at high risk in processing cancer-relevant information (Erblich et al. 2003). This study used a version of the classic Stroop task to investigate cognitive processing of cancer-related information. The Stroop task involves naming, quickly and accurately, the color of ink in which listed words appear. Delays or errors in naming the color are interpreted as resulting from cognitive interference introduced by the meaning of the words themselves. The study included women who had a family history of breast cancer (at least one first-degree relative affected) and women who had no family history. The modified Stroop task involved presenting lists of words that were related to cancer (e.g., *malignant*), cardiovascular disease (e.g., *coronary*), general threats (e.g., *nervous*), or were positive (e.g., *holiday*), or neutral (e.g., *furniture*).

The researchers found that for cancer-related words only, color-naming response latencies were significantly longer and errors were significantly more common for the women with a family history of breast cancer relative to those with no family history (Erblich et al. 2003). This difference in cognitive processing of cancer-related words is believed to reflect excessive vigilance by high-risk individuals toward cancer-related stimuli in general. Excessive vigilance toward specific, threatening stimuli is known to increase distress and interfere with information processing (Bower 1981). Thus, these findings have implications for the processing of complex information that women at high risk for breast cancer often encounter regarding cancer surveillance and prevention. Erblich and colleagues note that, in other areas of inquiry, interventions directed at specific worries have improved cognitive processing, suggesting a route toward treatment. However, statistical analyses revealed that the elevated levels of general distress, cancer-specific distress, and risk perception that were evident in the group of women with a family history of breast cancer in this study did not account for the differences found in their cognitive processing of cancer-related words. Women at high risk may differ in other ways, however, that can affect the way they process information. For example, women with a family history of breast cancer have been found to be more physiologically reactive than other women in response to laboratory stressors (Valdimarsdottir et al. 2002). This intriguing area of study requires extension to more naturalistic settings to determine the relevance of the findings detected in the laboratory to contexts involving critical exchanges of information, such as cancer risk counseling and genetic counseling.

Women whose family histories of breast (and other) cancers are so extensive that they are indicative of a likely hereditary influence now have the opportunity to undergo genetic testing to determine if they carry a mutation associated with an extremely high likelihood of developing breast (and ovarian) cancer. Psychosocial researchers have grappled with understanding the potential psychosocial risks and benefits of such testing. Potential benefits include relief in learning that one does not carry a deleterious mutation, which may also play a role in childbearing decisions or assist in understanding the cancer risk of offspring (Croyle et al. 1997). Even if one learns that one does carry a mutation, this can provide a sound basis for critical health care decisions such as whether or not to undergo prophylactic mastectomy (Botkin et al. 2003). Potential drawbacks of testing include distress at learning that one has tested positive for a mutation, guilt at learning that one has tested negative for mutation, conflicts among family members about whether to be tested, and strains among those who receive dissimilar test results (Biesecker et al. 1993; Biesecker 1997).

Not surprisingly, for women who decide to undergo testing, levels of anxiety increase soon after learning that they carry a mutation and decrease for women who do not. However, even among those without a mutation, having a sister who carries a mutation is associated with increased anxiety (Lodder et al. 2001). The first long-term follow-up studies of mutation carriers are now producing results which indicate that levels of distress 5 years after learning that one carries a mutation are predicted by pre-testing levels of worry about cancer, communication difficulties with family members, having young children, having lost a family member to cancer, and greater perception of risk (van Oostrom et al. 2003). However, women contemplating genetic testing report that being a member of a high-risk family is more distressing than the prospect of undergoing testing and those who anticipate the most distress may decline genetic testing (Coyne et al. 2003).

Either bilateral prophylactic mastectomy, often with breast reconstruction, or simple surveillance is an option for those who test positive for a mutation. Although women who opt for prophylactic surgery have higher distress after genetic testing than those who opt for surveillance or test negative, in the long-term, their levels of distress decline, most likely due to a reduction in fears of developing cancer (Lodder et al. 2002; van Oostrom et al. 2003). As suggested by cognitive dissonance theory, which predicts that individuals who voluntarily choose to undergo a procedure will typically not regret the results, long-term follow-up studies indicate that women are generally satisfied with the procedure despite declines in body image and sexual functioning over the same time period (van Oostrom et al. 2003).

TREATMENT DECISION-MAKING

A consensus conference was convened by the National Institutes of Health (NIH) in 1990 to review evidence on the efficacy of surgical treatments for breast cancer. It concluded that for many patients with early-stage disease, the combination of breast-conserving surgery, which removes only the tumor with a margin of normal tissue, plus radiation therapy is an appropriate option because of its equivalent survival to mastectomy, which removes the entire breast (NIH 1991). Long-term results from two randomized trials recently provided further evidence that breast-conserving surgical techniques when combined with radiotherapy are as effective as mastectomy in terms of survival for early-stage breast cancer (Fisher et al. 2002; Veronesi et al. 2002). The consensus conference also deemed breast-conserving treatment preferable because it preserves the breast and is thus less disruptive to body image. Indeed, dozens of studies have confirmed that body image is superior for women treated with this less invasive surgical technique (Moyer 1997). However, the two procedures differ in additional ways that are prioritized differently by different women. These include cost, the rate of disease recurrence in the primary affected breast, exposure to radiation, and length of treatment and recovery (Lantz et al. 2002). Meyerowitz and Hart found great diversity in women's views about the importance of body image in treatment preferences for breast cancer: "Some women criticize a lack of attention to body image and disfigurement and other women are offended by a focus on women's bodies" (Meyerwitz and Hart 1995, 78). Preferences are shaped by individual and sociocultural beliefs about the breast, its relationship to sexuality and body image, and the importance of body integrity (Lee et al. 2000; Ward et al. 1989).

Although there has been an increase in the adoption of breast-conserving surgery, concerns have been raised by demographic and regional disparities in its use (Albain et al. 1996; Gilligan et al. 2002; Polednak 2002). It is not clear whether such differences reflect genuine patient preferences (Gilligan et al. 2002). The proportion of women with breast cancer who should receive breast-conserving surgery is unknown (Ganz 1992), but its use should be based upon women being informed about the availability of breast-conserving treatment and its appropriateness in their particular case (Morrow 2002). Determining the appropriate amount and type of information has proven difficult, however. Promising decision aids have been developed using audiotapes and interactive CD-ROMs that assist in conveying this information clearly (Molenaar et al. 2001; Sawka et al. 1998).

Commonly cited research has found that that having input into one's choice of surgical treatment for breast cancer is related to better subsequent adjustment as indicated by lower anxiety, depression, and fear of recurrence, regardless of whether mastectomy or breast-conserving treatment was chosen (Morris and Royle 1987, 1988). However, these studies were limited because of their small sample sizes and the fact that having a choice of treatment was confounded with the type of treatment: All of the participants who were not given a choice of surgery were treated with mastectomy. A study in a larger sample without this limitation found that having input into one's choice of surgical treatment predicted greater satisfaction with one's medical treatment, but not lower psychological distress (Moyer and Salovey 1998). Other investigators have emphasized the importance of distinguishing between desire for information and desire for taking responsibility in decision-making (Fallowfield 2001).

TREATMENT SIDE EFFECTS

Although surgery and radiation therapy have painful and disconcerting side effects, the nausea and vomiting that can accompany chemotherapy are particularly debilitating. This concern has become more important as systemic adjuvant therapy involving Tamoxifen, combination chemotherapy, hormonal therapy, or a combination of these has become a dominant approach even for early-stage breast cancer patients (Hudis 2003). Anti-emetic medications are useful for some but not all patients, may provide only limited relief, and have side effects of their own. Anticipatory nausea, where simply thinking about or being exposed to cues reminiscent of chemotherapy administration makes one feel nauseated, as well as food aversions, are frustrating and uncomfortable side effects. Reducing such symptoms is important for maintaining patients' quality of life and increases the likelihood that patients will be able to continue to eat nutritiously and successfully adhere to their prescribed chemotherapy regimen

Researchers familiar with principles of learning have provided insights toward understanding the conditioned nature of side effects associated with cancer chemotherapy. From this perspective, these anticipatory symptoms develop when previously neutral stimuli in the environment, including the tastes of food, become associated with the nausea related to chemotherapy, and then come to elicit nausea and vomiting themselves (Andrykowski et al. 1988; Carey and Burish 1988; Montgomery and Bovbjerg 1997). Counter-conditioning approaches, where principles of learning are applied to reduce the association between nausea-inducing drug administration and benign aspects of the environment, show promise and can overcome the limitations of anti-emetic medications. One such approach is the overshadowing or "scapegoat" approach. This involves pairing the series of chemotherapy infusions with diverse, salient and unfamiliar, but pleasant, flavors, such as haw or elderberry juice drinks. Because of their novelty and strength, these flavors overshadow and diminish the associations formed with other stimuli in the environment. Preliminary work with this approach in small samples has shown only nonsignificant trends toward reducing anticipatory nausea and post-treatment nausea compared to control groups (Stockhorst et al. 1998). Nevertheless, this type of intervention deserves further attention because it is non-invasive, inexpensive, acceptable to patients, and without adverse effects.

Exacerbations of nausea and vomiting associated with cancer chemotherapy are also believed to result in part from psychological stress (Carey and Burish 1988). Thus, techniques designed to reduce stress, including hypnosis, progressive muscle relaxation (PMRT), guided imagery (GI), and systematic desensitization, have been used with some success (Burish and Tope 1992). For instance, one investigation compared standard anti-emetic treatment with PMRT and GI delivered either by a professional therapist, a volunteer therapist, or professionally produced audiotapes for treatment-related side effects in a group of breast, gynecologic, hemotologic, and lung cancer patients (Carey and Burish 1987). PMRT and GI delivered by a professional therapist reduced symptoms relative to the three other treatments in terms of patients' emotional distress and physiological arousal, and increased food intake. Levels of nausea did not differ among the groups but were initially low, suggesting that they were unlikely to be reduced further by the intervention. Although audiotapes were not found to be more effective than professional therapists, participants reported some positive features of the audiotapes such as privacy and blocking out sounds from the clinic. The authors of this study suggest that the effectiveness of audiotaped instruction PMRT and GI might be enhanced if preceded by a session with a therapist who explained instructions clearly and corrected initial difficulties.

Finally, correlational studies have documented an association between breast cancer patients' expectations about nausea and actual levels of anticipatory nausea that develop during chemotherapy. These studies indicate that such expectations have a unique effect on anticipatory nausea over and above the impact of other factors, including prior history of chemotherapy-related nausea and levels of distress (Montgomery and Bovbjerg 2001). This suggests that focusing on expectations could enhance current interventions that address psychological stress.

An often overlooked side effect of treatment for breast cancer is lymphedema. Damage to the lymphatic system from removal of axillary lymph nodes or from radiation therapy makes one vulnerable to developing this condition. Lymphedema is an abnormal collection of excessive tissue proteins, edema, chronic inflammation, and fibrosis in the arm and torso on the treated side (International Society of Lymphology 2003). Individuals with lymphedema experience swelling, pain, numbness, a loss of mobility, hardening and ulceration of the skin, and increased susceptibility to infection (Swirsky and Nannery 1998). Lymphedema usually occurs immediately after surgery, but can develop months or even years later. The reported incidence of lymphedema ranges from 6% to 30% (Petrek and Heelan 1998).

Little attention has been devoted to the psychosocial and functional impact of lymphedema. However, there are indications that lymphedema interferes significantly with quality of life (Dorval et al. 1998). Because lymphedema can occur at a point when cancer patients have completed their treatment and feel that they are on the road to recovery, its development can rekindle distress regarding the illness (Swirsky and Nannery 1998). The symptoms of lymphedema affect multiple facets of functioning. Arm and hand swelling can be difficult to conceal, even more than the loss of a breast. Some patients have problems with activities that involve lifting, gripping, and fine motor coordination (Passik et al. 1993). Moreover, pain and discomfort may exacerbate psychological distress, and sexual, physical and social dysfunction (Carter 1997; Passik et al. 1995).

Taking every step possible to avoid the onset of lymphedema is important. Because the condition is chronic, once it has developed managing the condition requires a great deal of time and effort; and resources for treatment, such as lymphedema therapists, are limited or unavailable in some areas. The suggested precautionary measures for women treated surgically for breast cancer include: avoiding infection, injury, pressure, or heat to the involved arm, being careful with vigorous activity, using caution when shaving the underarm area, keeping one's skin in good condition, maintaining one's ideal weight, and wearing a support garment or bandages when traveling by airplane (Burt and White 1999; Thiadens 1997).

Despite the dire consequences of developing lymphedema and the value of prevention, many patients report not having received information regarding either the possibility of lymphedema and arm problems or precautions they could take (Maunsell et al. 1993; Woods 1993). The optimal means to facilitate awareness of lymphedema are unknown. Many of the precautions are fairly simple to understand and adopt. For instance, if a patient about to undergo treatment for breast cancer is made aware that she should avoid injections, intravenous lines, or blood pressure cuffs on the arm on the treated side, and that bracelets are available to alert medical personnel to this fact, such measures may not be difficult for her to implement. However, other preventative measures include adaptations that may interfere to a greater extent with daily activities, such as not carrying heavy loads or avoiding repetitive arm motions. Developing strategies that help a woman implement and integrate these behavioral changes into her lifestyle may require more time, creativity, and support. Other helpful activities, such as self lymph massage and performing special exercises following breast cancer surgery, involve learning and practicing fairly complex sequences of behavior.

Although the precautions recommended to avoid lymphedema are extensive, the life changes required to alleviate lymphedema and maintain improvements are even more challenging. Although there is no standard treatment, reduction and control of lymphedema involves a comprehensive system of draining by a trained therapist, scrupulous skin cleansing, bandaging, exercise, and wearing a compression garment. Such a program is time-consuming and can interfere with other areas of functioning. Moreover, wearing bandages or a compression garment may make one feel self-conscious and lead to decreased social activity (Passik et al. 1993).

Some women could benefit from psychological and practical intervention to support them in coping with and managing lymphedema in addition to physical rehabilitation and pain management (Dennis 1993; Miller 1992; Passik et al. 1995). Although some psychiatrists and psychologists treat individuals with this condition and there are lymphedema support groups, developing professionally-led educational and supportive workshops or group meetings, with the input of physical therapists, lymphedema therapists, and psychotherapists, represents an underutilized opportunity for intervention.

COPING WITH BREAST CANCER

Although research has extensively documented the negative psychosocial impact of breast cancer, studies are beginning to focus on the observation that women also report positive outcomes of the breast cancer experience (Andrykowski et al. 1996; Cordova et al. 2001; Petrie et al. 1999; Taylor et al. 1984). The notion that positive life changes can develop following difficult transitions such as being diagnosed with a life-threatening illness has been called *post-traumatic growth* (Tedeschi and

Calhoun 1996). Cordova et al. found that compared to healthy participants (who rated changes since a matched point in time), women with breast cancer endorsed more positive changes since their diagnoses in relating to others, spirituality, and appreciation of life. In this study, the extent of posttraumatic growth in those with breast cancer was positively associated with participants' income, their perceived level of life threat due to their cancer, how much they had spoken to others about their breast cancer experience, and the length of time since their diagnosis. Further research has distinguished among the constructs *posttraumatic growth* (positive change resulting from struggling with a major life crisis), *benefit finding* (being able to identify benefit in adversity), and *positive reappraisal* (using benefit-related information as a coping strategy) in breast cancer patients (Sears et al. 2003). This work found that positive reappraisal predicted future posttraumatic growth, positive mood, and superior perceived physical health. Investigators recommend that therapeutic approaches which capitalize on posttraumatic growth (Antoni et al. 2001) could be beneficial but caution that expecting positive changes or pressuring patients to engage in positive thinking is inappropriate (Cordova et al. 2001).

Although disease-related factors are considered to be the most important determinants of cancer course and survival, researchers have hypothesized that psychological factors may also affect cancer progression (Epping-Jordan 1994). A biobehavioral model of cancer stress has been proposed whereby psychological and behavioral responses to stress influence biological processes and, perhaps, health outcomes (Andersen et al. 1994). Prior research had suggested that patients who engage in a "fighting spirit" rather than succumbing to feelings of helplessness or hopelessness have more positive outcomes in terms of cancer recurrence or survival (Greer 1990; Morris 1992). Accordingly, interventions were directed at bolstering this intrepid stance toward one's disease. Many breast cancer patients internalized the popular cultural value of "positive thinking" (Wilkinson and Kitzinger 2000). However, a recent comprehensive, systematic review of this research finds that there is insufficient evidence to conclude that coping styles (including fighting sprit, helplessness-hopelessness, denial, and avoidance) are related to cancer recurrence or survival (Petticrew 2002). One reason, according to Petticrew, is the existence of methodological limitations in studies investigating the impact of coping styles. For instance, other important predictors of cancer progression or survival are often not accounted for. Petticrew also found evidence of publication bias: studies which found benefits of coping styles used smaller samples of cancer patients than studies which found no effect. This suggests that smaller studies that contradicted these findings may have simply gone unpublished.

SUPPORTIVE INTERVENTIONS FOR BREAST CANCER PATIENTS

Psychosocial researchers and clinicians have been instrumental in developing and evaluating supportive treatments for breast cancer patients. The types of interventions developed to improve quality of life for people diagnosed with breast cancer are diverse and often multifaceted. Some resemble psychotherapeutic approaches used for treating psychological symptoms, such as group cognitive-behavioral therapy or psychodynamic psychotherapy. However, other, varied approaches have been tested in recent investigations, including a 10-week group cognitive-behavioral stress management intervention (Antoni et al. 2001), brief problem-focused or emotion-focused psycho-educational workshops (Rosberger et al. 2002), a nurse-administered intervention to enhance self-care self-efficacy (Lev et al. 2001), a 12-week complementary and alternative medicine support intervention (Targ and Levine 2002), and an intervention especially for younger women that used a problem-solving approach (Allen et al. 2002). Reviews of this area indicate that most interventions for cancer patients have been developed for and tested in breast cancer patients and that a variety of approaches are beneficial in terms of treatment- and disease-related symptoms and emotional and functional adjustment (Devine and Westlake 1995; Meyer and Mark 1995; Smith and Stullenbarger 1995; Trijsburg et al. 1992). Some of the challenges that remain for psychosocial researchers and clinicians involve determining the useful components of multidimensional treatments that have been found to be effective and finding ways to usefully implement fairly extensive and time-consuming interventions in community settings to the individuals who are most in need of them.

Psychologists have also alerted us to the potential limitations of aspects of psychosocial interventions long assumed to be beneficial. For instance, descriptive and correlational research show that emotional support, where one feels comfortable discussing worries and concerns with another person, is a process that cancer patients desire and benefit from, but there is a lack of evidence that interventions involving peer discussion with other cancer patients are beneficial (Helgeson and Cohen 1996). Theoretically, peer discussion groups are meant to encourage positive feelings toward oneself and increase self esteem by providing an environment of caring and acceptance, validating feelings through sharing, and encouraging cancer patients to feel less alone and unique in their experience. However, researchers have noted several ways in which peer discussion could have deleterious consequences. These include: group members raising uncomfortable or fear-arousing topics; alarm over group members who are not doing well; group interaction reinforcing one's identity as a member of a stigmatized group; group discussion breaking down protective defense mechanisms; and emotional support provided by members of such groups being perceived as "artificial" and thus not being as effective as that which comes from members of naturally occurring social networks (Helgeson and Cohen 1996). Similarly, in a previous, influential review of studies examining how cancer patients and other threatened groups satisfy their affiliative and informational needs, Taylor and Lobel (1989) showed that cancer patients seek contact with individuals whom they perceive as more fortunate. Participation in a peer discussion group may not be beneficial, therefore, if it exposes a woman with breast cancer to others doing poorly psychologically or physically.

Helgeson and colleagues directly tested the effects of a peer discussion intervention and a psychoeducational intervention for women with early-stage breast cancer (Helgeson et al. 2001a). Their study addressed some of the methodological shortcomings of prior work in this area by randomly assigning participants to groups, including a no-treatment control group, and recruiting a large enough sample to form multiple discussion groups for each treatment type to avoid conclusions based on the individual dynamics of one particular group. The interventions were also designed to be conducive to implementation outside of the research context by being short-term and delivered by oncology nurses and social workers who normally conduct support groups. The psychoeducational intervention was designed to reduce confusion and foster a sense of control over breast cancer by providing information about the disease and treatment and some methods for coping with problems like limited arm motion after surgery. The peer discussion intervention focused on expressing feelings and sharing experiences in a warm and accepting atmosphere. A third intervention group combined peer discussion and education, and in the control group, no intervention was provided.

Results indicated that at both 6 months and 3 years following the 8-week intervention there were clear benefits for the education intervention compared to the interventions that involved peer discussion or the control group (Helgeson et al. 1999, 2001b). Indeed, at 6 months, women in the peer discussion groups experienced an increase in intrusive and avoidant thoughts about their illness whereas those in the education group experienced a decrease in these symptoms. Although the treatment group differences declined over time, even after 3 years, women in the education-only group had greater vitality and physical functioning and less pain. The authors explained their findings by noting that the education intervention enhanced self-esteem and body image; they hypothesized that the information provided to patients helped them feel more competent and enabled them to perform day-to-day activities more readily. The negative outcomes found for peer discussion were consistent with Taylor and Lobel's (1989) earlier work: extended direct contact with individuals who, although at the same stage of breast cancer, had higher numbers of positive lymph nodes or more extreme chemotherapy side effects, was most likely alarming (Helgeson et al. 2001a). Alternatively, for peer discussion groups to be effective, a longer or more intense intervention than the one tested may be necessary (Helgeson et al. 2001b).

An additional possibility is that the success of an intervention is determined by the individual and situational characteristics of a breast cancer patient. As evidence, Helgeson and colleagues found that women with initially low levels of emotionally supportive resources benefited from all of the interventions whereas women who had low levels of personal resources such as feelings of control and certainty over their illness, self-esteem, and body image benefited most from the education-only intervention (Helgeson et al. 2000). Patients with a more controllable situation might benefit from problem-focused interventions, and those with worse prognosis and a less controllable situation might benefit more from emotion-focused approaches (Helgeson et al. 2001b). Furthermore, patients coping with early stages of the disease may require different types of assistance than those coping with other challenges.

Much debate surrounds the possibility that psychological interventions might extend the length of time that individuals with cancer survive (Cunningham et al. 1998, 1999; Fox 1998a, 1998b, 1999; Goodwin et al. 1999; Kraemer and Spiegel 1999; Spiegel et al. 1998). A well-known study by Spiegel and colleagues found that women with metastatic breast cancer who participated in a year-long weekly supportive-expressive group therapy intervention survived an average of 18 months longer than women who did not receive the intervention (Spiegel et al. 1989). However, a recent replication did not find a similar survival advantage (Goodwin et al. 2001). The relationship between psychological distress and disease course is complex (Spiegel 1996). Processes affected by psychosocial interventions that could conceivably affect somatic resistance to cancer include health-related behavior, treatment adherence, and hormonal, immunologic, and autonomic nervous system function (Andersen 2001; Andersen et al. 1994; Spiegel 2001).

An explanation for the inconsistency in this literature is supported by the observation that only a minority of the cancer patients involved in such interventions respond by making major changes, for instance, in their health related behavior or outlook. Cunningham and others (2000) found that among a group of 22 metastatic breast, colon, rectal, or pancreatic cancer patients who were motivated to undergo a year of weekly group therapy, longer survival was characterized by a constellation of psychological and cognitive factors that the authors termed "involvement with psychological self-help work." These factors were abstracted from analyses of therapy process notes, written homework assignments, and individual interviews. They included: the ability to act and change (e.g., lack of avoiding challenges); willingness to initiate changes (e.g., an intrinsic interest in exploring new behaviors); application to self-help work (e.g., amount and nature of self-help work); relationships with others (e.g., relations with the therapy group); and quality of experience (e.g., peace of mind). One factor, appraisal of threat, was not related to length of survival. These findings were particularly interesting and illuminating because a randomized trial conducted by the same researchers that randomly assigned metastatic breast cancer patients to an intervention designed to prolong their survival found no salutary effects on disease progression compared to controls (Cunningham et al. 1998). The authors assert that comparisons of group means in such trials where individuals are actively recruited and randomized may obscure the effects of a small number of highly involved patients by their inclusion with a majority of relatively less involved participants.

END-OF-LIFE ISSUES

Different periods in the course of being diagnosed and treated for breast cancer pose different challenges and difficulties. The end of life has received little attention in breast cancer patients. The end of life may present important problems such as coping with impending loss, as well as physical disability, deterioration, and fatigue. Recently, a long-term study carefully documented the course of distress symptoms in women with metastatic breast cancer until their death (Butler et al. 2003). This investigation indicated that, in the period before death, there was a significant elevation in mood disturbance, symptoms of trauma, and pain. This was accompanied by a decrease in the ability to experience positive states of mind. This spike occurred over and above any background levels of distress that participants were experiencing throughout the time that they were coping with metastatic breast cancer. These findings are important because they highlight the particular supportive needs of women with breast cancer at this point in disease progression and the need for specialized clinical interventions. The authors suggested that particular issues that should be dealt with included worries about death and dying, concerns about leaving dependent children and other loved ones, the increasing physical and cognitive disabilities that may accompany disease progression, and possible resultant deterioration in one's social environment.

CONCLUSION

The future of psycho-oncology involves challenges in three areas: clinical care, education and training, and research (Holland 1998). Psychosocial researchers and clinicians devoting their efforts toward improving the lives of breast cancer patients have important roles to play in evaluating the effectiveness of interventions, training future researchers and clinicians, and improving the quality and focus of research (Gruman and Convissor 1998). It is important to acknowledge also the ways in which breast cancer patients and advocates themselves have been important in making this possible. Through focusing attention on the disease, making clear the priorities and concerns of breast cancer patients, participating in research and in peer review, and successfully exerting pressure for increased funding, they have been important partners in providing the impetus and means for the field of psychosocial oncology to meaningfully address the difficulties of being at risk for or experiencing breast cancer.

Anne Moyer is Assistant Professor of Psychology at Stony Brook University and Marci Lobel is Associate Professor of Psychology at Stony Brook University. Anne Moyer was supported by a seed grant from the State University of New York at Stony Brook and Marci Lobel was supported by National Institutes of Health Grant R01HD39753 during the preparation of this chapter.

REFERENCES

Albain, K. S., S.R. Green, A.S. Lichter, L.F. Hutchins, W.C. Wood, I.C. Henderson, J.N. Ingle, J. O'Sullivan, C.K. Osborne, and S. Martino. 1996. Influence of patient characteristics, socioeconomic factors, geography, and systemic risk on the use of breast-sparing treatment in women enrolled in adjuvant breast cancer studies: an analysis of two intergroup trials. *Journal of Clinical Oncology* 14: 3009-3017.

Allen, S.M., A.C. Shah, A.M. Nezu, C.M. Nezu, D. Ciambrone, J. Hogan, and V. Mor. 2002. A problem-solving approach to stress reduction among younger women with breast carcinoma: a randomized controlled trial. *Cancer* 94: 3089-3100.

Andersen, B. L. 2001. A biobehavioral model for psychological interventions. In *Psychosocial Interventions for Cancer Patients,* ed. A. Baum and B.L. Anderson, 119-129. Washington, DC: American Psychological Association.

Andersen, B. L., J.K. Kiecolt-Glaser, and R. Glaser. 1994. A biobehavioral model of cancer stress and disease course. *American Psychologist* 49: 389-404.

Andrykowski, M. A., S.L. Curran, J.L. Studts, L. Cunningham, J.S. Carpenter, P.C. McGrath, D.A. Sloan, and D.E. Kenady. 1996. Psychosocial adjustment and quality of life in women with breast cancer and benign breast problems: A controlled comparison. *Journal of Clinical Epidemiology* 49: 827-834.

Andrykowski, M. A., Jacobsen, P. B., Marks, E., Gorfinkle, K., Hakes, T. B., Kaufman, R. J., Currie, V. E., Holland, J. C., and Redd, W. H. 1988. Prevalence, predictors, and course of anticipatory nausea in women receiving adjuvant chemotherapy for breast cancer. *Cancer,* 62: 2607-2613.

Antoni, M. H., J.M. Lehman, K.M. Kilbourn, A.E. Boyers, J.L. Culver, S.M. Alferi, S.E. Yount, B.A. McGregor, P.L. Arena, S.D. Harris, A.A. Price, and C.S. Carver. 2001. Cognitive-behavioral stress management intervention decreases the prevalence of depression and enhances benefit finding among women under treatment for early-stage breast cancer. *Health Psychology* 20: 20-32.

Biesecker, B.B. 1997. Psychological issues in cancer genetics. *Seminars in Oncology Nursing* 13: 129-134.

Biesecker, B. B., M. Boehnke, K. Calzone, D.S. Markel, J.E. Garber, F.S. Collins, and B.L. Weber. 1993. Genetic counseling for families with inherited susceptibility to breast and ovarian cancer. *Journal of the American Medical Association* 269: 1970-1974.

Botkin, J. R., K.R. Smith, R.T. Croyle, B.J. Baty, J.E. Wylie, D. Dutson, A. Chan, H.A. Hamann, C. Lerman, J. McDonald, V. Venne, J.H. Ward, and E. Lyon. 2003. Genetic testing for a BRCA1 mutation: Prophylactic surgery and screening behavior in women 2 years post testing. *American Journal of Medical Genetics* 118A: 201-209.

Bower, G. H. 1981. Mood and memory. *American Psychologist* 36: 129-148.

Burish, T.G. and D.M. Tope. 1992. Psychological techniques for controlling the adverse side effects of cancer chemotherapy: Findings from a decade of research. *Journal of Pain and Symptom Management* 7: 287-301.

Burt, J. and G. White. 1999. *Lymphedema: A Breast Cancer Patient's Guide to Prevention and Healing.* Alemeda, CA: Hunter House Publishers.

Butler, L.D., C. Koopman, M.J. Cordova, R.W. Garlan, S. DiMiceli, and D. Spiegel. 2003. Psychological distress and pain significantly increase before death in metastatic breast cancer patients. *Psychosomatic Medicine* 65: 416-426.

Carey, M.P. and T.G. Burish. 1988. Etiology and treatment of the psychological side effects associated with cancer chemotherapy: A critical review and discussion. *Psychological Bulletin* 104: 307-325.

———— 1987. Providing relaxation training to cancer chemotherapy patients: A comparison of three delivery techniques. *Journal of Consulting and Clinical Psychology* 55: 732-737.

Carter, B.J. 1997. Women's experiences of lymphedema. *Oncology Nursing Forum* 24: 875-882.

Cordova, M.J., L.L. Cunningham, C.R. Carlson, and M.A. Andrykowski. 2001. Posttraumatic growth following breast cancer: A controlled comparison study. *Health Psychology* 20: 176-185.

Coyne, J.C., L. Kruus, M. Racioppo, K.A. Calzone, and K. Armstrong. 2003. What do ratings of cancer-specific distress mean among women at high risk of breast and ovarian cancer? *American Journal of Medical Genetics* 116A: 222-228.

Croyle, R.T., K.R. Smith, J.R. Botkin, B. Baty, and J. Nash. 1997. Psychological responses to BRCA1 mutation testing: Preliminary findings. *Health Psychology* 16: 63-72.

Cunningham, A.J., C.V. Edmonds, G.P. Jenkins, H. Pollack, G.A. Lockwood, and D. Warr. 1998. A randomized controlled trial of the effects of group psychological therapy on survival in women with metastatic breast cancer. *Psychooncology* 7: 508-517.

Cunningham, A.J., C.V. Edmonds, and G.A. Lockwood. 1999. A careful investigation of an important phenomenon. *Psychooncology* 8: 364-366.

Cunningham, A.J., C.V. Edmonds, C. Phillips, K.I. Soots, D. Hedley, and G.A. Lockwood. 2000. A prospective, longitudinal study of the relationship of psychological work to duration of survival in patients with metastatic cancer. *Psychooncology* 9: 323-339.

Daly, M.B., C.L. Lerman, E. Ross, M.D. Schwartz, C.B. Sands, and A. Masny. 1996. Gail model breast cancer risk components are poor predictors of risk perception and screening behavior. *Breast Cancer Research and Treatment* 41: 59-70.

Dennis, B. 1993. Acquired lymphedema: A chart review of nine women's responses to intervention. *American Journal of Occupational Therapy* 47: 891-899.

Devine, E.C. and S.K. Westlake. 1995. The effects of psychoeducational care provided to adults with cancer: Meta-analysis of 116 studies. *Oncology Nursing Forum* 22: 1369-1381.

Dorval, M., E. Maunsell, L. Deschenes, J. Brisson, and B. Masse. 1998. Long-term quality of life after breast cancer: Comparison of 8-year survivors with population controls. *Journal of Clinical Oncology* 16: 487-494.

Epping-Jordan, J.E., B.E. Compas, and D.C. Howell. 1994. Predictors of cancer progression in young adult men and women: Avoidance, intrusive thoughts, and psychosocial symptoms. *Health Psychology* 13: 539-547.

Erblich, J., G.H. Montgomery, H.B. Valdimarsdottir, M. Cloitre, and D.H. Bovbjerg. 2003. Biased cognitive processing of cancer-related information among women with family histories of breast cancer: Evidence from a cancer stroop task. *Health Psychology* 22: 235-244.

Fallowfield, L. 2001. Participation of patients in decisions about treatment for cancer. *British Medical Journal* 323: 1144.

Fisher, B., S. Anderson, J. Bryant, R.G. Margolese, M. Deutsch, E.R. Fisher, J.H. Jeong, and N. Wolmark. 2002. Twenty-year follow-up of a randomized trial comparing total mastectomy, lumpectomy, and lumpectomy plus irradiation for the treatment of invasive breast cancer. *New England Journal of Medicine* 347: 1233-1241.

Fox, B.H. 1999. Clarification regarding comments about a hypothesis. *Psychooncology* 8: 366-367.

——— 1998a. A hypothesis about Spiegel et al.'s 1989 paper on psychosocial intervention and breast cancer survival. *Psychooncology* 7: 361-370.

———1998b. Rejoinder to Spiegel et al. *Psychooncology* 7: 518-519.

Ganz, P.A. 1992. Treatment options for breast cancer - beyond survival. *New England Journal of Medicine* 326: 1147-1149.

Gilligan, A.M., R.T. Kneusel, R.G. Hoffmann, A.L. Greer, and A.B. Nattinger. 2002. Persistent differences in sociodemographic determinants of breast conserving treatment despite overall increased adoption. *Medical Care* 40: 181-189.

Goodwin, P.J., M. Leszcz, M. Ennis, J. Koopmans, L. Vincent, H. Guther, E. Drysdale, M. Hundleby, H.M. Chochinov, M. Navarro, M. Speca, and J. Hunter. 2001. The effect of group psychosocial support on survival in metastatic breast cancer. *New England Journal of Medicine* 345: 1719-1726.

Goodwin, P.J., K.I. Pritchard, and D. Spiegel. 1999. The Fox guarding the clinical trial: Internal vs. external validity in randomized studies. *Psychooncology* 8: 275.

Greer, S., T. Morris, K. Pettingale, and J. Haybittle. 1990. Psychological response to cancer and 15-year outcome. *Lancet* 335: 49-50.

Gruman, J.C. and R. Convissor. 1998. Bridging the gap between research, clinical practice, and policy. In *Psycho-oncology*, ed. J.C. Holland, 1173-1176. New York: Oxford University Press.

Helgeson, V.S. and S. Cohen. 1996. Social support and adjustment to cancer: Reconciling descriptive, correlational, and intervention research. *Health Psychology* 15: 135-148.

Helgeson, V. S., S. Cohen, R. Schulz, and J. Yasko. 2001a. Group support interventions for people with cancer: Benefits and hazards. In *Psychosocial interventions for cancer*, ed. A. Baum and B.L. Anderson, 269-286. Washington, DC: American Psychological Association.

——— 2001b. Long-term effects of educational and peer discussion group interventions on adjustment to breast cancer. *Health Psychology* 20: 387-392.

——— 2000. Group support interventions for women with breast cancer: Who benefits from what? *Health Psychology* 19: 107-114.

——— 1999. Education and peer discussion group interventions and adjustment to breast cancer. *Archives of General Psychiatry* 56: 340-347.

Holland, J.C. 1998. Societal views of cancer and the emergence of psycho-oncology. In *Psycho-oncology*, ed. J.C. Holland, 3-15. New York: Oxford University Press.

Hudis, C.A. 2003. Current status and future directions in breast cancer therapy. *Clinical Breast Cancer* 4, Suppl 2: S70-75.

International Society of Lymphology. 2003. The diagnosis and treatment of peripheral lymphedema. Consensus document of the International Society of Lymphology. *Lympholog,* 36: 84-91.

Kraemer, H. and D. Spiegel. 1999. Cunning but careless: Analysis of a non-replication. *Psychooncology* 8: 273-275.

Lantz, P.M., J.K. Zemencuk, and S.J. Katz. 2002. Is mastectomy overused? A call for an expanded research agenda. *Health Services Research* 37: 417-431.

Lee, M.M., S.S. Lin, M.R. Wrensch, S.R. Adler, and D. Eisenberg. 2000. Alternative therapies used by women with breast cancer in four ethnic populations. *Journal of the National Cancer Institute* 92: 42-47.

Lerman, C., M. Daly, C. Sands, A. Balshem, E. Lustbader, T. Heggan, L. Goldstein, J. James, and P. Engstrom. 1993. Mammography adherence and psychological distress among women at risk for breast cancer. *Journal of the National Cancer Institute* 85: 1074-1080.

Lerman, C., K. Kash, and M. Stefanek. 1994. Younger women at increased risk for breast cancer: perceived risk, psychological well-being, and surveillance behavior. *Journal of the National Cancer Institute Monographs* 16: 171-176.

Lev, E.L., K.M. Daley, N.E. Conner, M. Reith, F. Cristina, and S.V. Owen. 2001. An intervention to increase quality of life and self-care self-efficacy and decrease symptoms in breast cancer patients. *Scholarly Inquiry for Nursing Practice* 15: 277-294.

Lodder, L., P.G. Frets, R.W. Trijsburg, E.J. Meijers-Heijboer, J.G. Klijn, H.J. Duivenvoorden, A. Tibben, A. Wagner, C.A. van der Meer, A.M. van den Ouweland, and M.F. Niermeijer. 2001. Psychological impact of receiving a BRCA1/BRCA2 test result. *American Journal of Medical Genetics* 98: 15-24.

Lodder, L., P.G. Frets, R.W. Trijsburg, E.J. Meijers-Heijboer, J.G. Klijn, C. Seynaeve, A.N. van Geel, M.M. Tilanus, C.C. Bartels, L.C. Verhoog, C.T. Brekelmans, C.W. Burger, and M.F. Niermeijer. 2002. One-year follow-up of women opting for presymptomatic testing for BRCA1 and BRCA2: Emotional impact of the test outcome and decisions on risk management surveillance or prophylactic surgery. *Breast Cancer Research and Treatment* 73: 97-112.

Maunsell, E., J. Brisson, and L. Deschenes. 1993. Arm problems and psychological distress after surgery for breast cancer. *Canadian Journal of Surgery* 36: 315-320.

Meyer, T.J. and M.M. Mark. 1995. Effects of psychosocial interventions with adult cancer patients: A meta-analysis of randomized experiments. *Health Psychology* 14: 101-108.

Meyerowiz, B.E. and S. Hart. 1995. Women and cancer: Have assumptions about women limited our research agenda? In *The Psychology of Women's Health: Progress and Challenges in Research and Application,* ed. A.L. Stanton and S.J. Gallant, 51-84. Washington, DC: American Psychological Association.

Miller, L.T. 1992. *Recovery in Motion: An Exercise Program to Assist in the Management of Upper Extremity Lymphedema.* Philadelphia, PA: L.T. Miller.

Molenaar, S., M.A. Sprangers, E.J. Rutgers, E.J. Luiten, J. Mulder, P.M. Bossuyt, J.J. van Everdingen, P. Oosterveld, and H.C. de Haes. 2001. Decision support for patients with early-stage breast cancer: Effects of an interactive breast cancer CD-ROM on treatment decision, satisfaction, and quality of life. *Journal of Clinical Oncology* 19: 1676-1687.

Montgomery, G.H. and D.H. Bovbjerg. 2001. Specific response expectancies predict anticipatory nausea during chemotherapy for breast cancer. *Journal of Consulting and Clinical Psychology* 69: 831-835.

———— 1997. The development of anticipatory nausea in patients receiving adjuvant chemotherapy for breast cancer. *Physiology and Behavior* 61: 737-741.

Morris, J. and G.T. Royle. 1988. Offering patients a choice of surgery for early breast cancer. *Social Science and Medicine* 26: 583-585.

———— 1987. Choice of surgery for early breast cancer: Pre-and post-operative levels of clinical anxiety and depression in patients and their husbands. *British Journal of Surgery* 74: 1017-1019.

Morris, T.P., K. Pettingale, and J. Haybittle. 1992. Psychological response to cancer diagnosis and disease outcome in patients with breast cancer and lymphoma. *Psychooncology* 1: 105-114.

Morrow, M. 2002. Rational local therapy for breast cancer. *New England Journal of Medicine* 347: 1270-1271.

Moyer, A. 1997. Psychosocial outcomes of breast-conserving surgery versus mastectomy: A meta-analytic review. *Health Psychology* 16: 284-298.

Moyer, A. and P. Salovey. 1998. Patient participation in treatment decision-making and the psychological consequences of breast cancer surgery. *Women's Health* 4: 103-116.

National Institutes of Health. 1991. NIH consensus conference. Treatment of early-stage breast cancer. *Journal of the American Medical Association* 265: 391-395.

Passik, S., M. Newman, M. Brennan, and J. Holland. 1993. Psychiatric consultation for women undergoing rehabilitation for upper-extremity lymphedema following breast cancer treatment. *Journal of Pain Symptom Management* 8: 226-233.

Passik, S.D., M.L. Newman, M. Brennan, and R. Tunkel. 1995. Predictors of psychological distress, sexual dysfunction and physical functioning among women with upper extremity lymphedema related to breast cancer. *Psychooncology* 4: 255-263.

Petrek, J.A. and M.C. Heelan. 1998. Incidence of breast carcinoma-related lymphedema. *Cancer* 83, Suppl 12: 2776-2781.

Petrie, K.J., D.L. Buick, J. Weinman, and R.J. Booth. 1999. Positive effects of illness reported by myocardial infarction and breast cancer patients. *Journal of Psychosomatic Research* 47: 537-543.

Petticrew, M., R. Bell, and D. Hunter. 2002. Influence of psychological coping on survival and recurrence in people with breast caner: A systematic review. *British Medical Journal* 325: 1066-1075.

Polednak, A.P. 2002. Trends in, and predictors of, breast-conserving surgery and radiotherapy for breast cancer in Connecticut, 1988-1997. *International Journal of Radiation Oncology, Biology, Physics* 53: 157-163.

Rosberger, Z., L. Edgar, J.-P. Collet, and M.A. Fourneir. 2002. Patterns of coping in women completing treatment for breast cancer: A randomized controlled trial of Nucare, a brief psychoeducation workshop. *Journal of Psychosocial Oncology* 20: 19-37.

Sawka, C.A., V. Goel, C.A. Mahut, G.A. Taylor, E.C. Thiel, A.M. O'Connor, I. Ackerman, J.H. Burt, and E.H. Gort. 1998. Development of a patient decision aid for choice of surgical treatment for breast cancer. *Health Expectations* 1: 23-36.

Schwartz, M.D., C. Lerman, and B.K. Rimer. 2001. Psychosocial interventions for women at increased risk for breast cancer. In *Psychosocial Interventions for Cancer*, ed. A. Baum and B.L. Anderson, 287-304. Washington, DC: American Psychological Association.

Schwartz, M.D., B.K. Rimer, M. Daly, C. Sands, and C. Lerman. 1999. A randomized trial of breast cancer risk counseling: The impact on self-reported mammography use. *American Journal of Public Health* 89: 924-926.

Sears, S.R., A.L. Stanton, and S. Danoff-Burg. 2003. The yellow brick road and the emerald city: Benefit finding, positive reappraisal coping and posttraumatic growth in women with early-stage breast cancer. *Health Psychology* 22: 487-497.

Smith, M.C. and E. Stullenbarger. 1995. An integrative review and meta-analysis of oncology nursing research: 1981-1990. *Cancer Nursing* 18: 167-179.

Spiegel, D. 1996. Psychological distress and disease course for women with breast cancer: One answer, many questions. *Journal of the National Cancer Institute* 88: 629-631.

Spiegel, D. 2001. Mind matters - group therapy and survival in breast cancer. *New England Journal of Medicine* 345: 1767-1768.

Spiegel, D., J.R. Bloom, H.C. Kraemer, and E. Gottheil. 1989. Effect of psychosocial treatment on survival of patients with metastatic breast cancer. *Lancet* 2: 888-891.

Spiegel, D., H.C. Kraemer, and J.R. Bloom. 1998. A tale of two methods: Randomization versus matching trials in clinical research. *Psychooncology* 7: 371-375.

Stockhorst, U., J.A. Wiener, S. Klosterhalfen, W. Klosterhalfen, C. Aul, and H.J. Steingruber. 1998. Effects of overshadowing on conditioned nausea in cancer patients: An experimental study. *Physiology and Behavior* 64: 743-753.

Swirsky, J. and D.S. Nannery. 1998. *Coping With Lymphedema*. Garden City Park, NY: Avery Publishing Group.

Targ, E.F. and E.G. Levine. 2002. The efficacy of a mind-body-spirit group for women with breast cancer: A randomized controlled trial. *General Hospital Psychiatry* 24: 238-248.

Taylor, S.E., R. Lichtman, and J. Wood. 1984. Attributions, beliefs about control, and adjustment to breast cancer. *Journal of Personality and Social Psychology* 46: 489-502.

Taylor, S.E. and M. Lobel. 1989. Social comparison activity under threat: Downward evaluation and upward contacts. *Psychological Review* 96: 569-575.

Tedeschi, R.G. and L.G. Calhoun. 1996. The posttraumatic growth inventory: Measuring the positive legacy of trauma. *Journal of Trauma Stress* 9: 455-471.

Thewes, B., B. Meiser, K. Tucker, and V. Schnieden. 2003. Screening for psychological distress and vulnerability factors in women at increased risk for breast cancer: A review of the literature. *Psychology, Health, and Medicine* 8: 289-304.

Thiadens, S.R.J. 1997. *Eighteen Steps to Prevention for Upper Extremities*. San Francisco, CA: National Lymphedema Network.

Trijsburg, R.W., F.C. van Knippenberg, and S.E. Rijpma. 1992. Effects of psychological treatment on cancer patients: A critical review. *Psychosomatic Medicine* 54: 489-517.

Valdimarsdottir, H.B., S.G. Zakowski, W. Gerin, J. Mamakos, T. Pickering, and D.H. Bovbjerg. 2002. Heightened psychobiological reactivity to laboratory stressors in healthy women at familial risk for breast cancer. *Journal of Behavioral Medicine* 25: 51-65.

van Oostrom, I., H. Meijers-Heijboer, L.N. Ladder, H.J. Duivenvoorden, A.R. van Gool, C. Seynaeve, C.A. van der Meer, J.G. Klijn, B.N. van Geel, and C.W. Burger. 2003. Long-term psychological impact of carrying a BRCA1/2 mutation and prophylactic surgery: A 5-year follow-up study. *Journal of Clinical Oncology* 21: 3867-3874.

Veronesi, U., N. Cascinelli, L. Mariani, M. Greco, R. Saccozzi, A. Luini, M. Aguilar, and E. Marubini. 2002. Twenty-year follow-up of a randomized study comparing breast-conserving surgery with radical mastectomy for early breast cancer. *New England Journal of Medicine* 347: 1227-1232.

Ward, S., S. Heidrich, and W. Wolberg. 1989. Factors women take into account when deciding upon type of surgery for breast cancer. *Cancer Nursing* 12: 344-351.

Wilkinson, S. and C. Kitzinger. 2000. Thinking differently about thinking positive: A discursive approach to cancer patients' talk. *Social Science and Medicine* 50: 797-811.

Woods, M. 1993. Patient's perception of breast cancer-related-lymphedema. *European Journal of Cancer Care* 2: 125-128.

IV. BREAST CANCER IN THE CLASSROOM

CHAPTER TWELVE

HELEN RODNITE LEMAY

TEACHING ABOUT BREAST CANCER AND "COMMON HEALTH"

This chapter will bring together insights from a volume on incorporating HIV/AIDS into the university classroom, *Learning for our Common Health* (1999), with reflections on teaching about breast cancer and women's health. Although the juxtaposition may at first seem a bit odd, it reflects my actual experience with the Stony Brook Breast Cancer conference, and with the other academic activities associated with it. Our inquiry into breast cancer took place within a Women's Studies class, Women's Studies 401: Women and Medicine, which was at the same time the site of a collaboration with a New York City public high school, The Young Women's Leadership School of East Harlem. The Association of American Colleges and Universities (AAC&U), also the sponsors of the HIV/AIDS volume, supported this collaboration.

The subtitle of *Learning for Our Common Health* is *How an Academic Focus on HIV/AIDS Will Improve Education and Health,* and the authors devote a good deal of their effort to exploring the goals and ideals of education. These represent an appropriate point of departure for discussion of Women's Studies for this discipline has, since its inception, taken seriously pedagogical issues—why study women in society and culture? How do we define the aims of our teaching? What role do bodies play in history, in the classroom, in students' lives? These questions, basic to the Women's Studies classroom, are also prominent in the volume.

The AAC&U authors have set down basically two goals. First, they want to improve health understood in a large sense, and secondly they intend to work toward this improvement within the university setting, while strengthening liberal education. The two aims, they maintain, are inextricably interconnected. On a practical level, as David Burns points out, most of the professionals who will be affecting health care, either as direct practitioners or as community leaders, are trained in colleges and universities. Further, and most importantly, "colleges are also engaged in the important work of educating citizens" (Burns 1999, 8).

M.C. Rawlinson and S. Lundeen (eds.), The Voice of Breast Cancer in Medicine and Bioethics, 185-194.

Women's Studies 401 students certainly represented an appropriate group for influencing health care, for six of the nine undergraduates enrolled in my Women and Medicine seminar had clearly committed to medical careers, as had two of the part-time teaching assistants. Further, all had either completed or were well advanced in their science prerequisites. They had voluntarily enrolled in this elective course, largely because they believed that in one way or another it would advance their medical careers, and they were ready to think deeply about health issues.

Burns calls for universities to help students develop "an appreciation for human commonalities and differences, and...a good grasp of the democratic processes (the arts of citizenship) required to deliberate and achieve effective consideration in the public sphere" (Burns 1999, 6). Women's Studies 401 students probably had a head start on the first of these goals, because of the very international character of the class, typical of Stony Brook University. One student was born in Russia, one in Moldova, two in Nigeria, one in the Philippines, and one in Haiti. One was either born in China or first-generation Chinese, and the other two were from Long Island, New York, where Stony Brook University is located. Certainly the structure of the course encouraged them to question and deliberate, although democratic processes were not directly addressed.

Probably the most important point in this volume, made by almost all the contributors, is that the idea of health goes beyond the individual, hence the adjective "*common*" in the title. Richard Keeling points out that normally we think of health as "a biomedical quality possessed by individuals" and use modifiers for any other understanding of the word (public health, community health, mental health) (Keeling 1999, 65), and certainly that was the initial approach of our students to breast cancer. One saw herself as a "carrier" of the Breast Cancer gene, although she had no solid evidence of this (only a family history of "suspicious" mammograms), and others thought in terms of themselves, or family members, and their susceptibility to the disease. The course was designed to widen these perspectives by introducing historical, social and political analyses, and raising, as Keeling puts it "essential, deeper human questions about the self, relationships, community, culture—the obligations and responsibilities of individuals and societies" (ibid., 55).

This is a tall order for a seminar that will spend less than six weeks investigating breast cancer, and will then move on to other women's health topics, and integrate high school students into the discussion. William Cronon, who would, I believe, include this class in his call for "liberal" learning understood in the etymological sense—"education for human freedom, education for the fulfillment of human talent and human promise," approaches "the cultural construction of disease" through an examination of history, and that is precisely how we began (Cronon 1999, 38). Because we were interested not only in disease, but also in human bodies, and specifically in *women's* bodies, we began with discussion of female fertility goddesses, and read a number of chapters from Margaret Yalom's *History of the Breast* (1997). We considered "The Sacred Breast" and "The Erotic Breast," and juxtaposed these two concepts with reflection on a chapter from a La Leche manual written in 1958 (which was the one available when I gave birth in 1972), and a few readings on breast augmentation surgery and silicone implants. We were, of course, exploring what women's breasts meant in the past, and what they signify today. In this early part of the course we moved from an individual perspective to a larger one, always, however, coming back to our own experiences. In some ways we followed the precepts set down by Burns: 1) Begin with the self. 2) Move beyond the self. 3) Return to the self. 4) Repeat the process (Burns 1999, 10-11). This personal note became especially striking when one of the students told us in one of the first meetings that she had breast reduction surgery scheduled for spring break.

Cronon uses Charles Rosenberg's *The Cholera Years* (1987) to make the point that the same disease can appear very different in different eras. Although cholera was always tied to the same infectious agent, it was perceived as three distinct diseases in the epidemics of 1832, 1849, and 1866. At first an illness caused by bad air and bad atmosphere to which immoral people were particularly susceptible, cholera moved on to become a disorder caused by a germ, which could be controlled by quarantine, burning clothes of the infected, and cleaning up the water (Cronon 1999, 41). Breast cancer too, has been constructed differently throughout history. We read from Ellen Leopold's *A Darker Ribbon: Breast, Cancer, Women, and Their Doctors in the Twentieth Century* (2000) about the impact of religion on ideas of disease, the source of the taboo about breast cancer, the martyrdom of Saint Agatha (whose breasts were amputated), and the significance of breast cancer to women and their doctors in nineteenth-century Victorian society.

One particularly valuable section of this volume is comprised of the chapters entitled, "A Really Hideous Mutilation: The Radical Mastectomy in the Correspondence of a Breast Cancer Patient and Her Surgeon, William Stewart Halsted (1917-22)," and "A Little Private Hell: The Letters of Rachel Carson and Dr. George Crile, Jr. 1960-64." Reading this primary source material and comparing it with Rose Kushner's *Why Me? What Every Woman Should Know About Breast Cancer to Save Her Life* (1975) provided us with more than a sense of pre-feminist and post-feminist approaches to dealing with one's disease. It also gave us a feeling of engagement with the material, which Keeling characterizes as "the key to transformative education" (Keeling 1999, 72). The issues of the role of women in the family, privacy, truth telling, and individual responsibility for one's health care, raised in the voices of women struggling through a painful period of their lives, allowed us to reflect on some commonalities of women's experiences with disease.

Cronon lists a number of questions that arise from consideration of medical history. Among them are: What is the culture of medical expertise? What is the guild that possesses information defining the disease, and how does this expertise shape treatment? How does the cost of producing, distributing, and marketing new therapies, particularly drug treatments, reflect the political economy of the corporations that deliver these therapies to the marketplace (Cronon 1999, 43)? These issues were very much on our mind as we turned to our next readings from Barron Lerner's *The Breast Cancer Wars: Hope, Fear, and the Pursuit of a Cure in Twentieth-Century America* (2001). As we learned about the close ties between medical politics and the development of biometrics, radiation and the modified radical mastectomy, we realized just how interested members of the male medical guild were in professional advancement, and how heavily this weighed in their choice of treatment for women patients. When, later in the course, we read an essay by Jane S. Zones, "Profits from Pain: The Political Economy of Breast Cancer" (2000), we saw how costly new commodities led to profit for private companies, who exaggerated claims of benefit. We learned as well of research and treatment biases—e.g., length bias, which means that women whose tumors are discovered earlier appear to be living longer than women who are diagnosed at a later date; selection bias, which refers not only to preferential choice of subjects in a study, but also to elimination of participants from outcome statistics if they die during chemotherapy; and of doctors' overstatement of the benefits of chemotherapy.

Zones draws a sharp contrast between "the trend in breast cancer research…toward increasingly expensive and technical solutions," and the "public health perspective [that] calls for prioritizing research and programs that would eliminate the causes of this disease before it develops" (Zones 2000, 141). Her observation that "[i]n the twentieth century, public health preventive measures, including environmental, social, behavioral, and nutritional improvements, have had a far greater impact on survival than medical technologies, including penicillin and vaccination" (ibid., 142), coupled with the evidence she presents of corporate efforts to oppose these measures, take us back to the idea of common health that informs the AAC&U volume. While Keeling calls for "understanding the social and cultural contexts of health and health decisions, and allocating resources toward community-based, rather than purely individual interventions" (Keeling 1999, 55), Zones tells a story of pharmaceutical companies, who are producers of herbicides and pesticides, censoring printed material used in Breast Cancer Awareness month, which they sponsor. They focus on mammography, on examination of individual women, regardless of their demographic risk, instead of community action as the best protection against the disease.

As practitioners of the discipline of Women's Studies, not only do we examine the social and cultural contexts of heath in terms of the tension between individual and society, but more importantly, we feature in our analysis the variable of gender. Cronon acknowledges that, "the struggle against HIV, the struggle against AIDS, is also a struggle over questions…of the way gender is constructed in the culture" (Cronon 1999, 45), and this is no less true with breast cancer. Society prescribes certain roles for women, whose reactions to these instructions have consequences far beyond the individual. After Saint Agatha was punished for rejecting the sexual advances of a governor of the Roman empire by having her breasts amputated, and then died an agonizing death, her canonization emphasized the sanctity of passivity and suffering for women (Leopold 2000, 30). When breast cancer struck in the Victorian family and the wife and mother became incapable of carrying out her duties, the only way to deal with the terrible void was to hide it, and to blame the patient for her own failings.

Concealment and passivity are two of the themes depicted in Cherisse Saywell's study of representations of breast cancer in the British media (2000). During a three-year period (1995-1997), only two pictures out of 800 were of mastectomized breasts, even though breasts are omnipresent in the media—the mutilation of a sexualized part of the body is not for public display. The message that women are supposed to sacrifice themselves for God and family is evident in the plentiful accounts of healthy young women from "cancer-dense" families undergoing prophylactic double mastectomies in order to save themselves to raise their children, and of other women whose cancer was discovered during their pregnancy, who turned down treatment to save their unborn children. Saywell comments that "[i]n all of the mother-centered stories women were depicted using metaphors of sainthood and martyrdom" (Saywell 2000, 50).

Self-negation is not the only role prescribed for women, however. Certainly Matuschka, whose image on the cover of *The New York Times Magazine* in 1993 revealed her mastectomized chest, and Audre Lorde, who refused the pale pink prosthesis offered to her by a Reach to Recovery volunteer, followed a different path. Probably the topic that was most revealing to our class of societal messages given to women with breast cancer was breast reconstruction. We learned from Lerner that while to Lorde "reconstruction was an 'atrocity' that compounded the sins of a prosthesis," by the 1980s the operation was widely popular, desired by three out of five eligible women (Lerner 2001, 192-3). The tension between some feminists who situated reconstruction within a patriarchal culture that focused on an "impossible aesthetic" for the female breast, and others who argued that every woman had a right to do whatever she could to put the cancer experience behind her was echoed in our class discussions of breast augmentation, so evident in the club scene with which some students were quite familiar. This was a Women's Studies class in which some women did *not* classify themselves as "feminist," and embraced, rather than feeling oppressed by, contemporary American standards for female appearance.

It was especially instructive for us to read, then, some chapters from Susan Zimmerman's *Silicone Survivors: Women's Experiences with Breast Implants* (1998). The author reports that half of the women she interviewed were "thrilled" with their new breasts after surgery: "Once entrapped in bodies that seemed 'different' and 'abnormal,' these women saw their decision to receive breast implants as a liberating experience" (Zimmermann 1998, 73). The other half had very different perceptions. Well before any from either group became ill, twenty out of forty of the patients were angry. Although they felt more attractive and more sexually confident, they also expressed resentment. One woman, for example, stated: "I didn't feel good about feeling more sexual with the implants…I was really angry inside that I had had to put plastic bags filled with chemicals in my body in order for me to feel like I could do the Hoochie Koo on Saturday nights" (ibid., 74). Even the women in Nina Hallowell's study of women who had reconstruction after prophylactic mastectomy found it to be problematic: their bodies felt unnatural. Not only had their nipple sensation disappeared, but they also felt different while negotiating the world. They were afraid to hug other people, conscious that their "boobs" were "like a buffer" (Hallowell 2000, 171), and that physically they were not as they seemed.

Besides having surgery performed on their bodies to make them look attractive, or even normal, women who are suffering are often required to "put on a happy face." Lerner gives us an account of books and magazine articles that began to appear in the mid-to-late 1970s emphasizing the positive aspects of the breast cancer experience. Helga Sandburg Crile, wife of one of the most famous breast cancer surgeons and daughter of the poet Carl Sandburg, wrote an article for *McCall's* magazine in 1974 entitled, "Let a joy keep you" (Lerner 2001, 300). Marvella Bayh, whose husband was a United States Senator, published an autobiography describing the inspiration she received from a Reach to Recovery volunteer, and making note of many ways in which cancer had changed her life for the better (ibid., 300-301). These messages, too, have been subjected to criticism. Sharon Batt, for example, points out that, "Reach to Recovery falsifies the breast cancer experience by packaging it as a cosmetic mishap, only slightly more serious than a broken fingernail," and that "Look Good, Feel Better," the sister organization, "makes a fetish of looking 'normal'" (Batt 1988, 144). Batt recognizes that a woman who is undergoing chemotherapy might prefer taking a nap to putting on makeup, might need a shoulder to cry on instead of alienating those close to her by pretending things are fine.

Of course cultural messages for women are not uniform for all races and classes, nor do all have the same means to follow them. Among the questions listed by Cronon as worth investigating is how people who are differently positioned in society perceive their own vulnerability to disease, how they separate themselves from those who are more vulnerable, and how this sense of separation articulates class, gender, and other boundaries within the culture (Cronon 1999, 44). Robert Fullilove and Mindy Thompson Fullillove inform us in *Learning for Our Common Health* that, "the complexion of HIV/AIDS is increasingly black and brown," and they quote Jonathan Mann to the effect that as epidemics mature, the brunt often shifts to "those who were socially marginalized or discriminated against before the epidemic began" (Fullilove and Fullilove 1999, 107-108). Breast cancer is, of course, not an epidemic; nevertheless, it is experienced differently by different groups. Zillah Eisenstein in *Manmade Breast Cancers* (2001) writes of "Pluralized Environments in Black and White." Racism, she maintains, is expressed in societal disregard for environmental concerns. Cancer mortality rates are higher for blacks than for whites; air is filthier in black communities; environmental toxins increase according to poverty, and disproportionate numbers of blacks are poor. Poor communities have less access to medical diagnosis and treatment; "[r]ace, class, and health hazards combine" (Eisenstein 2001, 96). Anne Kasper studied urban poor women with breast cancer, and concluded that, "[t]he multiple and persistent features of poverty that precede and follow the women's breast cancer diagnosis and treatment are of greater consequence than whether or not they are insured" (Kasper 2000, 183). Delays in diagnosis and treatment, and compromised quality of care all weighed heavily in the disease experience. Yet, even in Finland, a country with universal health care, women in the lowest social class had a risk of death from breast cancer that was 1.3 times greater than women in the highest social class (188). Clearly, factors such as fear of loss of home and job, and simply not having enough to live on or to take care of one's loved ones take a toll on health and survival.

One prominent theme in both the HIV/AIDS and breast cancer movements has been social activism. In *Learning for our Common Health,* Ira Harkavy and Daniel Romer address this topic from the perspective of service learning (Harkavy and Romer 1999), however political activism does not, appropriately, figure in the university projects the authors describe. Ulrike Boehmer examines this area of politics in *The Personal and the Political* (2000). Subtitled *Women's Activism in Response to the Breast Cancer and AIDS Epidemics,* Boehmer's study maintains that the AIDS movement benefited from the experience of feminist and women's health movement activists, that women in ACT UP publicized the ways in which women with AIDS were "scapegoated and framed as carriers of the disease" (Boehmer 2000, 15). At the same time, AIDS served as an "enabler for the grassroots breast cancer movement in the 1990s" (ibid., 16), for the feminist strategies used in ACT UP served as a basis for that decade's activism. Boehmer includes in her analysis the factors of race, economic and social differences, disease status, and sexual orientation. She demonstrates that although AIDS activism caters to impoverished groups, whereas the cancer movement "thrives on white middle-class values, tools and resources" (ibid., 56), the processes and cultures of these two worlds have much in common.

Nora Kizer Bell introduces the topic of ethics in her essay in the AAC&U volume, "Learning About AIDS and Ethics in a Liberal Democracy." Bell makes the point that examining ethical issues raised by HIV disease seems to be "a natural forum for developing ethical reasoning and heightening moral sensitivities" (Kizer Bell 1999, 98). Surely the same is true for breast cancer, and our class included discussion of feminist bioethics. We learned from Susan Sherwin's seminal work, *No Longer Patient: Feminist Ethics and Health Care,* of the "importance of considering the ways in which medicine supports and participates in the complex systems of practices that constitute the oppression of women" (Sherwin 1992, 89). While most non-feminist writers, according to Sherwin, examine medical practices in isolation from their historical and political contexts, we were able to use her chapters to help us "consider ethical questions in a contextually-based framework" (ibid., 91). Sherwin cites Kathryn Morgan to the effect that we cannot apply such traditional concerns as informed consent and confidentiality to an analysis of cosmetic surgery, for example, without looking at the context of an industry situated in a society that presents to women the basic message that they are flawed, that they must fit the norms dictated by fashion editors. Keeling makes a similar point when he states that "[a] deeper analysis of health behavior...suggests that health and health decisions always occur in context—within a social and cultural framework experienced through traditions, customs, folkways, media messages, peer group norms, and economic realities" (Keeling 1999, 65). Mary Rawlinson explores this further in her forthcoming book, *Medicine: Science of the Individual.* As Rawlinson puts it: "[E]thics has less to do with following rules of adjudicating conflicts of rights, than in recognizing the conditions of inequality in which most ethical dilemmas arise" (Rawlinson forthcoming).

We ended this course by following, in a sense, Burns' prescription to return to the self. At the end, we focused on the "selves" of breast cancer patients. We read their accounts of making treatment decisions, including Myrna Gene's "Saying No to a Mastectomy—Twenty-Five Years Ago" (Gene 1998); their stories of "Overcoming Cancer with Diet" (Greenfield 1998); and the cry to her friends, "Do it now. Do it all. Live your Dreams," of Barbara, newly diagnosed, in *Cancer in Two Voices* (Butler and Rosenblum 1991, 13). I, as the teacher, turned to the selves of my students—worried, at the end, that I had taken a group of vibrant young women and a man and moved them into depression after six weeks of concentrating on suffering, injustice, and oppression. I cannot really say what happened when they turned to their own selves; I can only hope that they found within the power to "only connect," as Cronon and E.M. Forster put it, that they became "more aware of [their] connections...with other people and with the rest of the planet" and cognizant, as well, of "the obligations we have to use our knowledge and our power responsibly, generously, caringly" (Cronon 1999, 50).

Helen Rodnite Lemay is Distinguished Teaching Professor of History at Stony Brook University.

REFERENCES

Batt, Sharon. 1988. Perfect people: Cancer charities. In *The Politics of Women's Bodies*, ed. Rose Weitz, 137-146. New York: Oxford University Press.

Boehmer, Ulrike. 2000. *The Personal and the Political: Women's Activism in Response to the Breast Cancer and AIDS Epidemics.* Albany: SUNY Press.

Burns, William David. 1999. Learning for our common health. In *Learning for Our Common Health: How An Academic Focus on HIV/AIDS Will Improve Education and Health,* ed. William David Burns, 1-19. Washington, D.C.: Association of American Colleges and Universities.

Butler, Sandra and Barbara Rosenblum. 1991. *Cancer in Two Voices.* Duluth: Spinsters Ink.

Cronon, William J. 1999. HIV, health, and liberal education. In *Learning for Our Common Health: How An Academic Focus on HIV/AIDS Will Improve Education and Health,* ed. William David Burns, 33-51. Washington, D.C.: Association of American Colleges and Universities.

Eisenstein, Zillah. 2001. *Manmade Breast Cancer.* Ithaca: Cornell University Press.

Fullilove, Robert E. and Mindy Thompson Fullilove. 1999. Placing HIV/AIDS in perspective: A question of history. In *Learning for Our Common Health: How An Academic Focus on HIV/AIDS Will Improve Education and Health,* ed. William David Burns, 105-117. Washington, D.C.: Association of American Colleges and Universities.

Gene, Myrna. 1998. Saying no to a mastectomy—Twenty-five years ago. In *Women Confront Cancer: Making Medical History By Choosing Alternative and Complementary Therapies,* ed. Margaret J. Wooddell and David Hess, 91-102. New York: New York University Press.

Greenfield, Louise. 1998. Overcoming cancer with diet. In *Women Confront Cancer: Making Medical History By Choosing Alternative and Complementary Therapies,* ed. Margaret J. Wooddell and David Hess, 103-109. New York: New York University Press.

Hallowell, Nina. 2000. Reconstructing the body or reconstructing the woman: Perceptions of prophylactic mastectomy for hereditary breast cancer risk. In *Ideologies of Breast Cancer: Feminist Perspectives,* ed. Laura K. Pott, 153-180. New York: St. Martin's Press.

Harkavy, Ira and Daniel Romer. 1999. Service learning and HIV/AIDS prevention: Prospects for an integrated strategy. In *Learning for Our Common Health: How An Academic Focus on HIV/AIDS Will Improve Education and Health,* ed. William David Burns, 75-93. Washington, D.C.: Association of American Colleges and Universities.

Kasper, Anne S. 2000. Barriers and burdens: Poor women face breast cancer. In *Breast Cancer: Society Shapes an Epidemic,* 183-212. New York: St. Martin's Press.

Keeling, Richard P. 1999. HIV/AIDS in the academy: Engagement and learning in a context of change. In *Learning for Our Common Health: How An Academic Focus on HIV/AIDS Will Improve Education and Health,* ed. William David Burns, 53-73. Washington, D.C.: Association of American Colleges and Universities.

Kizer Bell, Nora. 1999. Learning about HIV/AIDS and ethics in a liberal democracy. In *Learning for Our Common Health: How An Academic Focus on HIV/AIDS Will Improve Education and Health,* ed. William David Burns, 95-103. Washington, D.C.: Association of American Colleges and Universities.

Kushner, Rose. 1975. *Why Me? What Every Woman Should Know About Breast Cancer to Save Her Life.* New York: New American Library.

La Leche League International. 1958. *The Womanly Art of Breastfeeding.* Franklin Park, Illinois: La Leche League International.

Leopold, Ellen. 2000. *A Darker Ribbon: Breast Cancer, Women, and Their Doctors in the Twentieth Century.* New York: Beacon Press.

Lerner, Barron. 2001. *The Breast Cancer Wars: Hope, Fear, and the Pursuit of a Cure in Twentieth-Century America.* New York: Oxford University Press.

Rawlinson, Mary C. Forthcoming. *Medicine: Science of the Individual.* New York: Springer.

Rosenberg, Charles. 1987. *The Cholera Years.* Chicago: University of Chicago Press.

Saywell, Cherise with Lisa Beattie and Lesley Henderson. 2000. Sexualized illness: The newsworthy body in media representations of breast cancer. In *Ideologies of Breast Cancer: Feminist Perspectives,* ed. Laura K. Pott, 37-62. New York: St. Martin's Press.

Sherwin, Susan. 1992. *No Longer Patient: Feminist Ethics and Health Care.* Philadelphia: Temple University Press.

Yalom, Marilyn. 1997. *A History of the Breast.* New York: Knopf.

Zimmermann, Susan. 1998. *Silicone Survivors: Women's Experience with Breast Implants.* Philadelphia: Temple University Press.

Zones, Jane S. 2000. Profits from pain: The political economy of breast cancer. In *Breast Cancer: Society Shapes an Epidemic*, 119-151. New York: St. Martin's Press.

CHAPTER THIRTEEN

TANFER EMIN-TUNC

THEORETICAL CONSIDERATIONS ON "READING" THE BREAST

Creating a breast cancer reading group is a challenging venture because at its core lies the conflict between body politics and academia. Such groups are usually designed to serve as vehicles through which members of a community can discuss, and become actively involved with, issues concerning women's health and the female body. However, because of the varying backgrounds and vantage points of the individuals who are attracted to such groups, they either have the potential to be profoundly rewarding experiences in which the members of the group learn from, and teach, one another, or dismal disappointments in which personal and political differences cannot be transcended to create a meaningful dialogue.

This essay will examine the theoretical considerations involved in creating a breast cancer reading group while taking into account some of the broader social issues surrounding breast cancer studies and women's health. It will focus on a group of students who, during the spring of 2002, participated in a breast cancer reading group at Stony Brook University, in Long Island, New York.[1] The group was composed of about fifteen freshmen, ten female and five male, who enrolled in the reading group because of personal and academic interests. About ten of the fifteen students planned on attending medical school after completing their undergraduate studies, and believed that examining women's health from a humanities perspective would be beneficial to their perception of disease. The remaining five students either had a personal stake in breast cancer (namely, they had family members who were breast cancer survivors) or were interested in the breast as a cultural object.

The main objective of the group was to achieve a deeper understanding of women's health issues by examining the incidence, treatment, and social perception of breast cancer. The readings, which were articles and excerpts drawn from a number of disciplines (namely, medicine, biology, sociology, economics, philosophy, psychology, and history), focused on the breast as an historical subject

M.C. Rawlinson and S. Lundeen (eds.), The Voice of Breast Cancer in Medicine and Bioethics, 195-201.

whose meaning and treatment has changed with shifting social contexts. This multidisciplinary approach not only permitted pedagogical flexibility, but also introduced many of the participants to academic areas outside of their majors. Moreover, it compelled students to consider alternative epistemologies and, in the process, perfect their critical reading, thinking, and analytic skills.

The readings also served as a preliminary step toward the more important, and more difficult, task of rethinking "patriarchal" knowledge in light of the new perspectives made available when women's experiences are taken as a valid starting point. This theoretical approach did not simply "insert" women into the broad context of the *human condition*. Rather, it sought to restructure participants' understanding of the world by emphasizing the value of a woman-centered epistemology which prioritizes the *female condition*. This distinctly feminist methodology not only complemented the central themes of the reading group (e.g., debunking the essentialist myth that "anatomy is destiny"), but also stimulated many fascinating discussions about the place of breast cancer in the broader context of women's history.

We began our examination of breast cancer by focusing on the epidemiological aspects of the disease. During the first session, students were asked to look at a map depicting the incidence of breast cancer in Long Island, New York.[2] Because a majority of the students were from Long Island, this was not necessarily a shocking exercise: many were already aware of the abnormally high rates of breast cancer in their hometowns because they either experienced breast cancer first hand (a mother, sister, aunt, grandmother, female cousin, or close acquaintance battled the disease) or they had friends whose family members were breast cancer survivors. The point of this exercise was not to merely illustrate to students a fact they already knew. Rather, it was an attempt to convey the notion that personal and local events are often microcosms for public and global phenomena.

With that understanding, students then began the complicated task of viewing the breast as an object with a significant history that could provide them with insight into modern perceptions of female illness, sexuality, and gender roles. We first focused on two works from the breast cancer canon: Marilyn Yalom's *A History of the Breast* (1997), and La Leche League International's *The Womanly Art of Breastfeeding* (1990). Both readings focused on the *healthy* breast as a part of the body with a distinct history that incorporated religious, sexual, maternal (i.e., gendered), commercial, and medical concepts. After reading excerpts from these two works, students began to realize that the breast is not simply a part of the female anatomy. Rather, it is an object, actively produced by a culmination of social forces which, since the time of the ancients, have endowed it with meaning and allowed it to be "read" like a text. As Elizabeth Grosz maintains, breasts, and their accompanying bodies, cannot

> be adequately understood as ahistorical, precultural, or natural objects in any simple way; it is not simply that the body is represented in a variety of ways according to historical, social, and cultural exigencies while it remains basically the same; these factors actively produce the body as a body of a determinate type. (Grosz 1994, x)

We then shifted gears and concentrated on the breast as a social construct—both literally and figuratively. Norma Jacobson's *Cleavage: Technology, Controversy and the Ironies of the Man-Made Breast* (2000) compelled the group members to use complex poststructuralist theory to grapple with the implications of aesthetically re-configuring the postmodern body. The aspiring medical students in the group found this reading particularly useful because of its descriptions of breast surgery, and its commentary on why women, with seemingly "normal" and "healthy" breasts, voluntarily choose to change their bodies. This reading proved to be an excellent transition into current media portrayals of the body, and the ways in which large and small breasted pop culture icons, such as Pamela Anderson and Gwyneth Paltrow respectively, have dealt with praise/criticism of their own objectified breasts.

Our discussion of the "diseased" breast began with two of the seminal works from early breast cancer studies, which, along with women's health, emerged as a women's studies sub-specialty in the 1970s. George Crile's *What Women Should Know About the Breast Cancer Controversy* (1973) provided students with a glimpse into the state of medical knowledge in the early 1970s, while Rose Kushner's *Why Me? What Every Woman Should Know About Breast Cancer to Save Her Life* (1975) allowed students to view the disease, and its medically sanctioned treatments, through the eyes of a woman who battled breast cancer. Laura Potts's edited collection *Ideologies of Breast Cancer: Feminist Perspectives* (2000) proved to be the perfect contemporary complement to Crile's and Kushner's works. Two essays within *Ideologies of Breast Cancer* had a particularly profound impact on the students: Cherise Saywell's "Sexualized Illness" and Nina Hallowell's "Reconstructing the Body or Reconstructing the Woman." Both traced the sexualization of the diseased breast since the 1970s, and the ways in which women are, in the new millennium, coached to deal with breast cancer. Namely, they are told that breast cancer should not be seen as a *life-threatening* disease but rather as a *life-altering* disease.

Barbara Ehrenreich's essay "Welcome to Cancerland: A Mammogram Leads to a Cult of Pink Kitsch" (2001) seemed to resonate strongly with all of the students, most likely because it put a "face" on breast cancer—one with which many of the students could identify.[3] Ehrenreich reminded many of the participants of their own mothers, sisters, aunts, cousins, and grandmothers—intelligent women who did not want to become victims of breast cancer and the multi-billion dollar industry that accompanies it. Tired of the paternalistic, profit-oriented corporate and medical establishments, Ehrenreich, an accomplished feminist scholar, set out to document her own experiences with the disease. These experiences included battles with physicians who "suggested" that she undergo post-surgery breast augmentation to make her feel more like a "woman" (and make her husband feel more like a "man"), and encounters with the "cult of pink kitsch." According to Ehrenreich, this cult "brainwashes" millions of women every year to buy pink ribbons, infantile pink teddy bears, and breast cancer Barbies, whose molded plastic bodies serve as the template for breast implantations (Ehrenreich 2001, 49).

Many students were shocked that they too had participated in this culture of pink kitsch, which uses the technique of pseudo-feminist empowerment through the consumption of material goods to reduce breast cancer patients to children. Almost all of the students had purchased pink breast cancer paraphernalia of some kind, and, before participating in the reading group, even advocated breast implants and the aesthetic redesigning of female bodies for objective pleasure. Ehrenreich's article led the students to numerous epiphanies not just about themselves, but also about the capitalist, media-oriented consumer society in which we are all forced to live. They began to realize that women's bodies, and the diseases that affect them, are to a certain extent socially and commercially constructed. They came to terms with the reality that breast cancer survivors are often not adequately informed about the excruciating pain and torment of the disease and are, instead, told of its imaginary aesthetic "benefits." The students were astonished to learn that oncology nurses and survivors usually do not describe the horrors of chemotherapy, but rather express the notion that chemo "smoothes and tightens the skin, and helps you lose weight…and when your hair [does] come back, it will be fuller, softer, easier to control, and perhaps a surprising new color" (Ehrenreich 2001, 49). Chemo also has "the potential to render you [stronger], prettier and younger post-treatment, providing of course, that you survive" (ibid.).

Our reading group concluded with a collage of personal narratives. Three of the most memorable accounts were "Patient No More" (Batt 1998) which focuses on breast cancer survivor Susan Batt and her struggle to have her voice heard within the medical community; Myrna Gene's "Saying No to a Mastectomy—Twenty-Five Years Ago" (Gene 1998) in which she tackles the social, and medical, pressures that force women to conform to false ideals of beauty; and "Confronting National Breast Policy" (Holleran 1998) in which Susan Holleran discusses her activism within the realm of breast cancer legislation. One student was so moved by the class discussions regarding these personal accounts that he persuaded his mother and her best friend, both breast cancer survivors, to speak directly to the class. Bringing breast cancer survivors into the classroom who, as Long Island residents, were members of the students' immediate community, not only helped the group members understand the practical aspects of living with such a dreadful disease, but also made them realize that because of where they live, they, and their family members, were all potential breast cancer patients.[4]

In short, all of these theoretical concepts and approaches (e.g., using readings from multiple disciplines, emphasizing a feminist, woman-centered epistemology, presenting local epidemiological data, and incorporating personal accounts into the reading group) allowed me, the group facilitator, to tackle the socially complex material that often accompanies a politically infused topic such as breast cancer. Moreover, these methodologies also encouraged students to move beyond private emotions to interpret the public world through a critical lens. While for some students the reading group represented an epiphany in terms of the way they perceived the female body, illness, and sexuality, for others, it served to express and validate their own burgeoning opinions of the health care system and the way in which it treats women. The reading group, in my opinion, was an enormous success, not only because of the significant personal and academic breakthroughs that occurred within those fifteen weeks, but, more importantly, because students learned the important lesson that any major crisis in life can be overcome with serious introspection, discussion and self-empowerment.

Tanfer Emin-Tunc received her Ph.D. in History from Stony Brook University in 2005. Her area of specialization includes the history of medicine and reproductive technologies.

NOTES

1. Please see the reading list provided at the end of the chapter which lists the required texts for the reading group.

2. "Breast Cancer Incidence by Zip Code, 1993-1997," *The New York Times*, April 16, 2000.

3. I thank Dawn Zebrowski for introducing us to this article and its implications.

4. For a detailed discussion of the high incidence of breast cancer among Long Island residents, see Dr. John S. Kovach's chapter in this volume.

REFERENCES

Batt, Susan. 1998. Patient no more. In *Women Confront Cancer*, ed. Margaret J. Wooddell and David Hess, 309-313. New York: New York University Press.

Crile, George, Jr. 1973. *What Women Should Know About the Breast Cancer Controversy*. New York: Pocket Books.

Ehrenreich, Barbara. 2001. Welcome to cancerland: A mammogram leads to a cult of pink kitsch. *Harper's Magazine*, November: 49.

Gene, Myrna. 1998. Saying no to a mastectomy—Twenty-five years ago. In *Women Confront Cancer*, ed. Margaret J. Wooddell and David Hess, 321-327. New York: New York University Press.

Grosz, Elizabeth. 1994. *Volatile Bodies: Toward a Corporeal Feminism*. Bloomington: Indiana University Press.

Hallowell, Nina. 2000. Reconstructing the body or reconstructing the woman. In *Ideologies of Breast Cancer: Feminist Perspectives*, ed. Laura K. Potts, 79-91. New York: St. Martin's Press.

Holleran, Susan. 1998. Confronting national breast policy. In *Women Confront Cancer*, ed. Margaret J. Wooddell and David Hess, 331-338. New York: New York University Press.

Jacobson, Norma. 2000. *Cleavage: Technology, Controversy and the Ironies of the Man-Made Breast*. New Brunswick: Rutgers University Press.

Kushner, Rose. 1975. *Why Me? What Every Woman Should Know About Breast Cancer to Save Her Life*. New York: New American Library.

La Leche League International. 1990. *The Womanly Art of Breastfeeding.* Chicago: La Leche League International.

Potts, Laura K., ed. 2000. *Ideologies of Breast Cancer: Feminist Perspectives.* New York: St. Martin's Press.

Saywell Cherise. 2000. Sexualized illness. In *Ideologies of Breast Cancer: Feminist Perspectives*, ed. Laura K. Potts, 64-77. New York: St. Martin's Press.

Wooddell, Margaret J. and David Hess, eds. 1998. *Women Confront Cancer*. New York: New York University Press.

Yalom, Marilyn. 1997. *A History of the Breast*. New York: Knopf.

READING LIST

Blum, Linda. 2000. *At the Breast: Ideologies of Breastfeeding and Motherhood in the Contemporary United States.* New York: Beacon Press.

Boehmer, Ulrike. 2000. *The Personal and the Political: Women's Activism in Response to the Breast Cancer and AIDS Epidemics.* Albany: State University of New York Press.

Butler, Sandra and Barbara Rosenblum. 1991. *Cancer in Two Voices*. San Francisco: Spinsters Book Co.

Crile, George, Jr. 1973. *What Women Should Know About the Breast Cancer Controversy.* New York: Pocket Books.

Ehrenreich, Barbara. 2001. Welcome to cancerland: A mammogram leads to a cult of pink kitsch. *Harper's Magazine*, November: 49.

Eisenstein, Zillah. 2001. *Manmade Breast Cancers.* Ithaca: Cornell University Press.

Jacobson, Norma. 2000. *Cleavage: Technology, Controversy and the Ironies of the Man-Made Breast.* New Brunswick: Rutgers University Press.

Kasper, Anne S. and Susan Ferguson, eds. 2000. *Breast Cancer.* New York: St. Martin's Press.

Kushner, Rose. 1975. *Why Me? What Every Woman Should Know About Breast Cancer to Save Her Life.* New York: New American Library.

La Leche League International. 1990. *The Womanly Art of Breastfeeding.* Chicago: La Leche League International.

Leopold, Ellen. 2000. *A Darker Ribbon: Breast Cancer, Women, and Their Doctors in the Twentieth Century.* New York: Beacon Press.

Lerner, Barron H. 2001. *The Breast Cancer Wars: Hope, Fear, and the Pursuit of a Cure in Twentieth-Century America.* New York: Oxford University Press.

Lorde, Audre. 1980. *The Cancer Journals.* Argyle, New York: Spinsters, Inc.

Patterson, James T. 1987. *The Dread Disease: Cancer and Modern American Culture.* Cambridge: Harvard University Press.

Potts, Laura K., ed. 2000. *Ideologies of Breast Cancer: Feminist Perspectives*. New York: St. Martin's Press.

Proctor, Robert. 1997. *Cancer Wars: How Politics Shapes What We Know and Don't Know about Cancer*. New York: Basic Books.

Sherwin, Susan, ed. 1998. *The Politics of Women's Health: Exploring Agency and Autonomy*. Philadelphia: Temple University Press.

———— 1992. *No Longer Patient: Feminist Ethics and Health Care*. Philadelphia: Temple University Press.

The New York Times. 2000. Breast cancer incidence by zip code, 1993-1997. April 16.

Weitz, Rose, ed. 1988. *The Politics of Women's Bodies*. New York: Oxford University Press.

Wooddell, Margaret J. and David Hess, eds. 1998. *Women Confront Cancer*. New York: New York University Press.

Yalom, Marilyn. 1997. *A History of the Breast*. New York: Knopf.

Zimmermann, Susan. 1998. *Silicone Survivors*. Philadelphia: Temple University Press.

CHAPTER FOURTEEN

SOFYA MASLYANSKAYA

RECENT DEVELOPMENTS IN BREAST CANCER RESEARCH

Response to Dr. Kovach's chapter

In his chapter, Dr. John S. Kovach, the Founding Director of the Cancer Institute of Long Island, describes gene expression analysis, which is a technique that can provide us with information about many different genetic patterns of breast cancer. In the past, all cancers of the breast were treated with the same protocol based on the staging of the disease and the time period in which the patients lived. The new developments will allow physicians to prescribe different treatment plans based on the patient rather than a disease category. These advancements relate to scientific understanding of genetic mutations and of their effects on the human body. Investigators would not have been able to obtain this new information without the cooperation of large numbers of patients, and Dr. Kovach also discusses the trials and difficulties encountered in the research proceedings. This essay will expand upon both the laboratory and clinical aspects of recent investigations.

Scientists' knowledge of developments of cancer relies on the techniques that have been used in the past. The initial idea that tumors arise from changes in somatic cells (all cells besides egg or sperm cells) originated in the early 1900s. The technology to test this hypothesis only became available in the early 1970s, which is when the formation of cancerous cells was related to actions of certain genes. The experiments that were originally done involved the transfer of the gene being tested into a recipient cell.

Each gene has one allele that comes from the mother's genetic information and another that comes from the father's. Recessive alleles are those alleles that have little or no effect on the phenotype (visible properties such as color or shape) when a contrasting allele is present. At the time of this study it became known that the allele for malignancy was recessive (Ponder 2001, 337).

Mutations and alterations in genes are some of the important causes of breast cancer. A mutation in a single gene is not enough to cause a cell to become

203

M.C. Rawlinson and S. Lundeen (eds.), *The Voice of Breast Cancer in Medicine and Bioethics*, 203-207.

cancerous. Breast cancer results from genetic and environmental factors leading to the accumulation of mutations; therefore, inheriting a genetic mutation doesn't guarantee that the individual will develop cancer. In the future, when all of the genes are identified and patterns are made it will allow doctors to choose the right treatment for individual breast cancer sufferers. There is a need to identify more susceptibility genes, because the few that are known only account for 15-20% of breast cancer that runs in families and less than 5% of all breast cancers (Nathanson et al. 2001, 552).

Two of the genes that have been identified as breast cancer susceptibility genes are BRCA1 and BRCA2, which are caretaker genes. They maintain the global genome stability. They make sure that there is no unplanned loss, duplication or rearrangement of chromosomal DNA. When the genome stability is compromised it allows the cell to go beyond normal restriction points and continue growing, eventually causing cancer (Boyer and Lee 2001, 358). BRCA1 is a large gene that is involved in DNA damage response while the BRCA2 gene is even larger and is involved in chromosome segregation. (Genes are carried on DNA which winds itself up inside chromosomes. Chromosomes are located inside the nucleus of almost every cell in the human body. During cell division the chromosomes are duplicated and then divided to produce two daughter cells. Each daughter cell contains a copy of the chromosomes that were in the original cell.) When the BRCA2 gene is damaged it prevents normal segregation of chromosomes and damages the cell cycle. Some defects in DNA repair result in cancer predisposition syndrome, which is active in cancer progression (Nathanson et al. 2001, 553).

There are a few theories on how the inactivation of the BRCA1 and BRCA2 genes progresses. One of them is that the inactivation of these genes could make the breast susceptible to the effects of estrogen-induced DNA damage, which will result in inefficient or error prone cells. Another one is that BRCA1 mutations will promote epithelial cell proliferation, which means that cells will keep reproducing. This type of knowledge could help treat people with mutations in BRCA1 and BRCA2 genes and also patients with sporadic breast cancer, which is non-genetic cancer. Few of the sporadic breast cancers are caused by mutations in the BRCA1 and BRCA2 genes (Boyer and Lee 2001, 358).

BRCA1 and BRCA2 genes are high-penetrance, which means that there is a large amount of individuals of a particular genotype (that is, possessing genetic information), that express its phenotypic effect. Since these genes account only for 33% of families with four or five cases of breast cancer, researchers say that low-penetrance genes might be responsible for a large fraction of these families.

There is a problem with isolating low-penetrance genes because they rarely produce multiple care families, i.e., those families that have several cases of early-onset breast cancer. Since large population-based studies are expensive and time-consuming, another approach has been evaluated. This involves using age of diagnosis in people who are carriers of BRCA1 and BRCA2 mutations and then associating genetic variants with significant differences in age diagnosis. Since there is relatively little information available about what genes can be low-penetrance, researchers define areas of the genome where these genes might be located as ones that are biologically plausible (Nathanson et al. 2001, 554). Right now the screening for breast cancer susceptibility genes relies on a gene-by-gene experimentation, but the identification of these genes has been accelerated since the Human Genome Project was completed in April 2003 (Ponder 2001, 339).

Even though breast cancer has one name it acts very differently depending on the patient, so researchers try to use genetic screening techniques to predict breast cancer outcomes in different patients. DNA arrays analyze a sample for the presence of a gene mutation to identify patterns of gene expression. The goal is to develop a risk-profile system for each person with high accuracy in order to estimate the patient's prognosis and best form of treatment (Ahr et al. 2002, 131).

There have been a few new types of monitoring that have identified patients who might not benefit from adjuvant therapy, which is therapy that assists in the prevention of recurrence, such as chemotherapy (Roumen 2002, 179). This type of research also provides valuable information, which could be used to individualize the treatments of breast cancer patients.

In the paper, "Identification of High Risk Breast-Cancer Patients by Gene Expression," Dr.Ahr and his colleagues of the Goethe University in Frankfurt, Germany, used gene expression analysis to identify high risk breast cancer patients. Upon the completion of the study in 2002, two groups of patients were designated class A and non-class A. Cluster analysis using DNA arrays technology allows parallel expression profiling of several thousand genes and classification of tumors into categories based on shared gene expression patterns. The patients who were placed in class A, based on their gene pattern, included a high proportion of patients with nodal-positive tumors. If a tumor is nodal-positive it is an indication that cancer cells have moved from the cells of the organ to the lymph nodes. Lymph nodes are the filters along the lymphatic system. Their job is to filter out and trap bacteria, viruses, cancer cells, and other unwanted substances, and to make sure they are safely eliminated from the body. Since lymph travels throughout the body it is a way for cancer to metastasize (move to a different part of the body). Class A also had a high proportion of patients with distant metastases at the time of diagnosis. Consistent data was collected and after a median of 23.5 months they found out that 11 out of the 22 participants from class A progressed to metastatic disease. In class A 9 out of 20 had recurrences, compared to 3 out of 27 of non-class A. Even though class A and non-class A contained similar numbers of nodal-positive tumors, progression was limited mainly to class A. Even though validation studies need to be done, this evidence suggests that tumors of class A represent cancers with a high risk of recurrence (Ahr et al. 2002, 132).

Future studies must combine these molecular methods with the tumor classification systems that have been used in the past in order to develop therapies that are specifically tailored for each patient (Ahr et al. 2002, 132). Even though these studies will go on for years and will be very costly, the benefits will be colossal. The tools that will be developed as a result will indicate whom to screen, and how this screening should be conducted. Preventative and therapeutic therapies will also be developed which should greatly decrease the mortality from breast cancer (Nathanson et al. 2001, 556).

In his chapter, Dr. Kovach explains that in order to achieve good results researchers need large amounts of tissue samples to be able to identify more patterns and do so accurately. Scientists could share samples in order to be doing similar research in different institutions and to be able to compare their data. Scientists need to form a network in order to be able to collaborate on this imperative project.

There is a determined struggle to get more women to enter into clinical trials. Females make up most of the participants in breast cancer studies because of the view of breast cancer as being a disease of the "female" breast. Breast cancer patients as well as healthy patients who are at a high risk for getting the illness don't like to give something for nothing. Women who know about their predisposition have a certain degree of expectation to be able to choose a form of intervention that would be appropriate. In a placebo-controlled trial some patients get a placebo pill (a pill that contains an inactive substance such as sugar) while others get the drugs that are being tested. In his article, "Recruitment of Women into Trials," J.R. Benson found that in one International Breast Intervention Study (IBIS), the refusal rate (i.e., refusal to participate in the trial) due to the utilization of a placebo, was highest amongst mutation carriers (Benson 2002).

Some scientists suggest that future prevention studies should avoid placebo groups. One of the ways in which a placebo group could be eliminated is by randomizing two different types of drugs. In such a trial two groups of patients are usually picked arbitrarily by a computer program and each group receives a particular drug. Another way of increasing participation in trials is by sending out personal invitations that contain information and explanations about the trial to prospective participants (Benson 2002, 164). The invitations, of course, would be sent out by physicians in order to retain patient confidentiality.

Even though additional tens or even hundreds of predisposing alleles need to be identified, the goal of genotypic profiling is attainable. As genes are identified, they will be tested in large populations to predict the cancer incidence (Ponder 2001, 341). Now that the Human Genome Project is complete, the knowledge will allow susceptible breast cancer genes to be identified more quickly and more precisely. Even though not all breast cancers are genetic, this could give insight to what happens in sporadic cancers. The research will allow future generations to classify therapies not only in terms of illnesses, but also in terms of different pathways of disease in different people. Different treatments have to be tested numerous times before they become widely used.

This testing cannot take place without wide participation in trials, since blood and tissue samples are needed for analysis. Patient resistance must, therefore, be addressed. The randomization described earlier is one modification to research that can result in greater participation. It is important that more medical, social, and environmental knowledge be communicated between doctors and laypeople, so that doctors understand what would draw more people into studies, and laypeople might recognize that their contributions are needed and welcome.

Sofya Maslyanskaya received her Bachelor of Science degree in Biochemistry from Stony Brook University in 2004. She is currently attending medical school at the State University of New York, Downstate.

REFERENCES

Ahr, Andfre, Thomas Karn, Christine Solbach, Taja Seiter, Klaus Strebhard, Uwe Holtrich, and Manfred Kaufmass. 2002. Identification of high risk breast-cancer patients by gene expression profiling. *The Lancet* 359, no. 9301(Jan 12): 131-132.

Benson, J.R. 2002. Recruitment of women into trials. *The Lancet* 359, no. 9301 (Jan 12): 164.

Boyer, Thomas G. and Wen-Hwa Lee. 2001. BRCA1 and BRCA2 in breast cancer. *The Lancet* 358, supp. 1 (Dec 22): 5.

Nathanson, Katherine L., Richard Wooster, and Barbara L. Weber. 2001. Breast cancer genetics: What we know and what we need. *Nature Medicine* 7 (May 1): 552-556.

Ponder, Bruce A.J. 2001. Cancer genetics. *Nature* 411 (May 17): 336-341.

Roumen, Rudi M.H. 2002. Changing paradigms in breast cancer. *The Lancet* 359, no. 9301 (Jan 12): 179.

Philosophy and Medicine

Philosophy and Medicine

21. G.J. Agich and C.E. Begley (eds.): *The Price of Health.* 1986
ISBN 90-277-2285-4
22. E.E. Shelp (ed.): *Sexuality and Medicine.* Vol. I: Conceptual Roots. 1987
ISBN 90-277-2290-0; Pb 90-277-2386-9
23. E.E. Shelp (ed.): *Sexuality and Medicine.* Vol. II: Ethical Viewpoints in Transition.
1987   ISBN 1-55608-013-1; Pb 1-55608-016-6
24. R.C. McMillan, H. Tristram Engelhardt, Jr., and S.F. Spicker (eds.): *Euthanasia and the Newborn.* Conflicts Regarding Saving Lives. 1987
ISBN 90-277-2299-4; Pb 1-55608-039-5
25. S.F. Spicker, S.R. Ingman and I.R. Lawson (eds.): *Ethical Dimensions of Geriatric Care.* Value Conflicts for the 21th Century. 1987   ISBN 1-55608-027-1
26. L. Nordenfelt: *On the Nature of Health.* An Action-Theoretic Approach. 2nd, rev. ed. 1995   ISBN 0-7923-3369-1; Pb 0-7923-3470-1
27. S.F. Spicker, W.B. Bondeson and H. Tristram Engelhardt, Jr. (eds.): *The Contraceptive Ethos.* Reproductive Rights and Responsibilities. 1987
ISBN 1-55608-035-2
28. S.F. Spicker, I. Alon, A. de Vries and H. Tristram Engelhardt, Jr. (eds.): *The Use of Human Beings in Research.* With Special Reference to Clinical Trials. 1988
ISBN 1-55608-043-3
29. N.M.P. King, L.R. Churchill and A.W. Cross (eds.): *The Physician as Captain of the Ship.* A Critical Reappraisal. 1988   ISBN 1-55608-044-1
30. H.-M. Sass and R.U. Massey (eds.): *Health Care Systems.* Moral Conflicts in European and American Public Policy. 1988   ISBN 1-55608-045-X
31. R.M. Zaner (ed.): *Death: Beyond Whole-Brain Criteria.* 1988
ISBN 1-55608-053-0
32. B.A. Brody (ed.): *Moral Theory and Moral Judgments in Medical Ethics.* 1988
ISBN 1-55608-060-3
33. L.M. Kopelman and J.C. Moskop (eds.): *Children and Health Care.* Moral and Social Issues. 1989   ISBN 1-55608-078-6
34. E.D. Pellegrino, J.P. Langan and J. Collins Harvey (eds.): *Catholic Perspectives on Medical Morals.* Foundational Issues. 1989   ISBN 1-55608-083-2
35. B.A. Brody (ed.): *Suicide and Euthanasia.* Historical and Contemporary Themes.
1989   ISBN 0-7923-0106-4
36. H.A.M.J. ten Have, G.K. Kimsma and S.F. Spicker (eds.): *The Growth of Medical Knowledge.* 1990   ISBN 0-7923-0736-4
37. I. Löwy (ed.): *The Polish School of Philosophy of Medicine.* From Tytus Chałubiński (1820–1889) to Ludwik Fleck (1896–1961). 1990
ISBN 0-7923-0958-8
38. T.J. Bole III and W.B. Bondeson: *Rights to Health Care.* 1991
ISBN 0-7923-1137-X

Philosophy and Medicine

39. M.A.G. Cutter and E.E. Shelp (eds.): *Competency*. A Study of Informal Competency Determinations in Primary Care. 1991   ISBN 0-7923-1304-6
40. J.L. Peset and D. Gracia (eds.): *The Ethics of Diagnosis*. 1992
                                                                  ISBN 0-7923-1544-8
41. K.W. Wildes, S.J., F. Abel, S.J. and J.C. Harvey (eds.): *Birth, Suffering, and Death*. Catholic Perspectives at the Edges of Life. 1992 [CSiB-1]
                                                   ISBN 0-7923-1547-2; Pb 0-7923-2545-1
42. S.K. Toombs: *The Meaning of Illness*. A Phenomenological Account of the Different Perspectives of Physician and Patient. 1992
                                                   ISBN 0-7923-1570-7; Pb 0-7923-2443-9
43. D. Leder (ed.): *The Body in Medical Thought and Practice*. 1992
                                                                  ISBN 0-7923-1657-6
44. C. Delkeskamp-Hayes and M.A.G. Cutter (eds.): *Science, Technology, and the Art of Medicine*. European-American Dialogues. 1993   ISBN 0-7923-1869-2
45. R. Baker, D. Porter and R. Porter (eds.): *The Codification of Medical Morality*. Historical and Philosophical Studies of the Formalization of Western Medical Morality in the 18th and 19th Centuries, Volume One: Medical Ethics and Etiquette in the 18th Century. 1993   ISBN 0-7923-1921-4
46. K. Bayertz (ed.): *The Concept of Moral Consensus*. The Case of Technological Interventions in Human Reproduction. 1994   ISBN 0-7923-2615-6
47. L. Nordenfelt (ed.): *Concepts and Measurement of Quality of Life in Health Care*. 1994 [ESiP-1]   ISBN 0-7923-2824-8
48. R. Baker and M.A. Strosberg (eds.) with the assistance of J. Bynum: *Legislating Medical Ethics*. A Study of the New York State Do-Not-Resuscitate Law. 1995
                                                                  ISBN 0-7923-2995-3
49. R. Baker (ed.): *The Codification of Medical Morality*. Historical and Philosophical Studies of the Formalization of Western Morality in the 18th and 19th Centuries, Volume Two: Anglo-American Medical Ethics and Medical Jurisprudence in the 19th Century. 1995   ISBN 0-7923-3528-7; Pb 0-7923-3529-5
50. R.A. Carson and C.R. Burns (eds.): *Philosophy of Medicine and Bioethics*. A Twenty-Year Retrospective and Critical Appraisal. 1997 ISBN 0-7923-3545-7
51. K.W. Wildes, S.J. (ed.): *Critical Choices and Critical Care*. Catholic Perspectives on Allocating Resources in Intensive Care Medicine. 1995 [CSiB-2]
                                                                  ISBN 0-7923-3382-9
52. K. Bayertz (ed.): *Sanctity of Life and Human Dignity*. 1996
                                                                  ISBN 0-7923-3739-5
53. Kevin Wm. Wildes, S.J. (ed.): *Infertility: A Crossroad of Faith, Medicine, and Technology*. 1996   ISBN 0-7923-4061-2
54. Kazumasa Hoshino (ed.): *Japanese and Western Bioethics*. Studies in Moral Diversity. 1996   ISBN 0-7923-4112-0

Philosophy and Medicine

Philosophy and Medicine

74. H.T. Engelhardt, Jr. and L.M. Rasmussen (eds.): *Bioethics and Moral Content: National Traditions of Health Care Morality*. Papers dedicated in tribute to Kazumasa Hoshino. 2002   ISBN 1-4020-6828-2

75. L.S. Parker and R.A. Ankeny (eds.): *Mutating Concepts, Evolving Disciplines: Genetics, Medicine, and Society*. 2002   ISBN 1-4020-1040-0

76. W.B. Bondeson and J.W. Jones (eds.): *The Ethics of Managed Care: Professional Integrity and Patient Rights*. 2002   ISBN 1-4020-1045-1

77. K.L. Vaux, S. Vaux and M. Sternberg (eds.): *Covenants of Life. Contemporary Medical Ethics in Light of the Thought of Paul Ramsey*. 2002
                                                        ISBN 1-4020-1053-2

78. G. Khushf (ed.): *Handbook of Bioethics: Taking Stock of the Field from a Philosophical Perspective*. 2003   ISBN 1-4020-1870-3; Pb 1-4020-1893-2

79. A. Smith Iltis (ed.): *Institutional Integrity in Health Care*. 2003
                                                        ISBN 1-4020-1782-0

80. R.Z. Qiu (ed.): *Bioethics: Asian Perspectives A Quest for Moral Diversity*. 2003 [ASiB-3]   ISBN 1-4020-1795-2

81. M.A.G. Cutter: *Reframing Disease Contextually*. 2003   ISBN 1-4020-1796-0

82. J. Seifert: *The Philosophical Diseases of Medicine and Their Cure*. Philosophy and Ethics of Medicine, Vol. 1: Foundations. 2004   ISBN 1-4020-2870-9

83. W.E. Stempsey (ed.): *Elisha Bartlett's Philosophy of Medicine*. 2004 [CoME-2]
                                                        ISBN 1-4020-3041-X

84. C. Tollefsen (ed.): *John Paul II's Contribution to Catholic Bioethics*. 2005 [CSiB-3]   ISBN 1-4020-3129-7

85. C. Kaczor: *The Edge of Life*. Human Dignity and Contemporary Bioethics. 2005 [CSiB-4]   ISBN 1-4020-3155-6

86. R. Cooper: *Classifying Madness*. A Philosophical Examination of the Diagnostic and Statistical Manual of Mental Disorders. 2005   ISBN 1-4020-3344-3

87. L. Rasmussen (ed.): *Ethics Expertise*. History, Contemporary Perspectives, and Applications. 2005   ISBN 1-4020-3819-4

88. M.C. Rawlinson and S. Lundeen (eds.): *The Voice of Breast Cancer in Medicine and Bioethics*. 2006   ISBN 1-4020-4508-5

springer.com